I0090432

Prenatal Nurturing & Nutrition:

A Critical Window of Opportunity to Embrace a Conscious Pregnancy

Madonna Igah-Okoro, PhD, MPH, BS

Copyright © Madonna Igah 2024

All Rights Reserved

All rights reserved. No part of this publication may be reproduced, distributed, or transmitted in any form or by any means, including photocopying, recording, or other electronic or mechanical methods, without the author's prior written permission, except in the case of brief quotations embodied in critical reviews and certain other non-commercial uses permitted by copyright law. For permission requests, please get in touch with the author.

Contents

Dedication i

Acknowledgements ii

About the Author iii

Introduction 1

Prenatal Nurturing & Nutrition 4

Session #1 4

Prenatal Nurturing & Nutrition 21

Session #2 21

Prenatal Nurturing & Nutrition 41

Session #3 41

Lesson Worksheets 56

Course Exam 59

Exam Answer Key 60

References 61

Presentation Slides 63

Dedication

In support of Prenatal Families Everywhere.

Acknowledgements

I would like to give particular mention to Cheri—gratitude and well wishes.

Also, I would like to heartily thank my ever-so-loving and inspiring family, Frank Maduka Igah Sr., Flora Obiageli Igah, Katherine Adanma Igah, Flora Ejeoma Igah, Roswitha Obiageli Igah, Frances Chiamaka Igah, Frank Maduka Igah Jr., Koby Zita Igah, husband Nnamdi Okoro, and very special thanks to my precious baby Divina.

About the Author

Madonna has been an educator for over 10 years now, leading general health/wellness and nutritional-based courses and programs.

Madonna is a content creator, a curriculum instructional designer/developer, and a course instructor. Madonna holds a Bachelor of Science degree in Biology Pre-Medicine, a Master of Public Health Management and Policy degree, and a PhD in Public Health Prevention Science.

Madonna is also a mother, by virtue of a successful natural and unmedicated labor and delivery. She is eternally grateful for her victorious water birth, and relentlessly amazed by her magnificent child--surely, a divine gift from the Most High.

Introduction

Welcome to Prenatal Nurturing and Nutrition (online OR in-person) course! This course was created by Madonna Igah, PhD, to meet the unique needs of expectant persons/couples. The course curriculum offers foundational knowledge and skills for cultivating a healthy pregnancy that excludes fetal maltreatment and further encourages nurturing techniques after childbirth. This guide uniquely includes a complete script, allowing for ease in delivering lessons, flexibility regarding who leads the lessons, and opportunity for individual reading/learning.

Effective Lesson Subject-Matters

- Instruction on the catchphrase "Prenatal Nurturing and Nutrition," as well as the importance of timely and comprehensive Prenatal Care.

- Instruction on pregnancy fears and hopes and communication with an unborn child.

- Instruction on mental, physical, emotional, spiritual, and social changes associated with pregnancy, pregnancy hormones, and relaxation activities.

- Instruction on maternal and fetal physical development.

- Instruction on proper prenatal nutrition.

- Instruction on the potential effects of substance use/abuse during the prenatal period.

- Lesson worksheets are included that will equip participants with the ability to recall and describe lesson instruction and continue active learning outside of class lectures. A post-examination that will allow for the assessment of participants' knowledge upon course completion is also included. In each lesson, participants have the opportunity to discuss class topics within small-group formats, i.e., breakout sessions. This will allow for the potential elimination of isolation through the strengthening of social networks, inclusive of persons having similar challenges. The course was constructed for both online and in-person applications.

Overarching Program Goal:

Recent research has shown how suboptimal prenatal care and conditions can alter the development of the unborn child and that issues can persist to early adulthood. Further, without prenatal educational programs, expecting persons may (either intentionally or unintentionally) engage in high-risk behaviors that have the potential to cause harm to themselves or to their unborn child. A meta-analysis of 142 papers examined the effects of various interventions relating to parental education in the prenatal and postnatal periods (Pinquart & Teubert, 2010). Child abuse/neglect was one of the focal outcomes assessed. Further, along with the outcome of child abuse/neglect, there were several other outcomes that are either directly or indirectly related to child abuse/neglect that the review reports on as well (including parenting skills, parental stress, health-promoting parental behavior, child development, parental psychological health, and couple adjustment). All of these outcomes mentioned were shown to have positive changes with the aforementioned interventions.

The primary goal of this program is to utilize interactive lessons to assist expecting women and their partners in establishing a paramount belief in themselves as parents who are nurturing and are capable decision-makers in fostering conditions that are conducive to optimal growth and development of the unborn child. For the best outcomes regarding children, it is necessary to provide informational support for parents prenatally.

Additional Program Goals:

- Increase Parental Resilience through enhancing skills regarding proper management of stress and a gained knowledge of successful functioning when faced with pregnancy challenges.
- Increase Social Connections by providing opportunities for parents to become acquainted through small-group discussions.
- Increase knowledge of child development through instruction on anatomical and physiological fetal and maternal development during the prenatal period.
- Help ensure that expecting parents and their unborn child are on a trajectory of positive and nurturing outcomes.

Disclaimer: All class content is for educational purposes only and does not substitute professional medical advice or consultations with healthcare professionals.

Today's Topics

- Welcome to Lesson 1 of Prenatal Class! (After Class opening & introductions); For today's lesson, we will discuss the importance of Prenatal Care, the meaning of Prenatal Nurturing and Nutrition, different pregnancy wishes and pregnancy concerns, and the significance behind connecting with your unborn baby.

Prenatal Care

- Prenatal care, simply put, is the care that a woman gets during her pregnancy. When most people think of prenatal care, they think of health procedures such as medical checkups and screening tests. These are typically included in Prenatal Care (in efforts to properly monitor mom and your baby throughout the entire pregnancy). However, Prenatal care can also include things like education (such as what we are doing here today) and counseling on how to handle the different periods and different aspects of your pregnancy.

- Be prepared to have ongoing conversations with different care providers. During prenatal visits with your doctor, you may be asked to discuss different issues such as your diet and physical activity level, screening tests you might need, and what to expect during labor and delivery.

- It is very important to start prenatal care as early as possible! The best possible situation would be to begin care before the pregnancy starts. More realistically, starting as early as possible means starting as soon as a woman knows or thinks she is pregnant.

- It is also very important to be consistent in going regularly for prenatal care treatments. This can help both moms and their babies to stay as healthy as possible. Regular care allows increased opportunity for your prenatal Healthcare Provider(s) to find and manage any pregnancy issues as soon as possible.

- Research shows that prenatal care makes a huge difference for a healthy pregnancy. Women who do not seek prenatal care are three times as likely to deliver a low birth-weight infant. Lack of prenatal care can also increase the risk of infant death. As you can see, your prenatal care is very important!

Prenatal Care Cont.

- There are a few things to consider when thinking about your Prenatal Care. Some of the more significant things include choosing the best Prenatal Care Provider, determining where you (plan) to Deliver Your Baby, understanding Prenatal Checkups, understanding Prenatal Tests, being aware of whether or not your pregnancy is considered High-Risk, and maintaining proper Prenatal Nutrition.

Choosing a Prenatal Care Provider

- You will need to have several appointments/interactions with your prenatal care provider before you birth your baby. You want to be sure that you choose a person that you are comfortable going on this prenatal journey with (such as a person that has a good reputation, and listens to you, and respects you). You should also find out if the doctor (or midwife) can deliver your baby in the way and place that you desire to give birth.

- A few Health care providers that care for women during pregnancy include Obstetricians, Family Practice Doctors, Midwives, and Doulas.

- **Obstetricians (otherwise known as OBs)** are medical doctors who specialize in the care of pregnant women and in delivering babies. OBs also have special training in surgery, so they are also able to perform a cesarean delivery (otherwise known as a C-section) as well. Women who have existing health issues or are at risk for pregnancy complications should see an obstetrician. In some instances, women with high-risk pregnancies may also need special care from a **maternal-fetal medicine specialist**.

- **Family practice doctors** are medical doctors who provide care for an entire family throughout all of the different stages of life. This can actually include care during pregnancy and delivery, as well as following birth. If you have a great relationship with your Family Practice Doctor and desire to seek their continued care during pregnancy and delivery, you may want to reach out to your doctor and discuss all of the possibilities. Keep in mind, however, that most family practice doctors cannot perform cesarean deliveries.

- **Certified nurse-midwife (CNM)** and **certified professional midwife (CPM)** are trained to provide both pregnancy and postpartum care. If you are a healthy woman and at low risk for problems during pregnancy, labor, and delivery, midwives may be a good option. CNMs are educated in both nursing and midwifery and typically practice in hospitals and birth centers. All midwives can provide expert care, counseling, and support to women and their families throughout the prenatal and postpartum periods. Also, all midwives should have a back-up plan (that includes assistance from an obstetrician) in case of a problem or emergency.

- A doula is a professional labor coach who provides unique support for women and their partners during the prenatal, labor, and delivery periods. For example, a doula may offer physical and emotional support that includes guidance on different breathing techniques, personal relaxation methods, helpful movement(s), and proper positioning. It is very possible for doulas and midwives to work together.

- Research has shown that continuous support from a doula during labor was linked to shorter labors and much lower use of pain medications, oxytocin (a hormone that helps labor to progress by stimulating uterine contractions), and cesarean delivery. If you desire support from a doula, make sure to check with your health insurance company to find out if they will cover the cost. You may also want to find out if your doula is certified by Doulas of North America (DONA) or another professional establishment.

- Ask around to get different view-points and opinions! For example, you can talk to your primary care doctor, friends, and family members for different provider recommendations. Ultimately, make sure that when you are making your choice, you are patient with yourself in taking different factors into consideration. Of course, some factors that are very important for some people may hold little or no importance for others. However, some examples of things that you may want to consider include a provider's reputation, personality, bedside manner, gender, age, office location (is it close to your home?), office hours, experience level, how phone consultations are handled, how after-hour calls are handled, whether you will always be seen by the same provider for appointments and delivery, who covers if the provider becomes unavailable, and where the delivery will likely take place. Don't be shy about making the best possible choice here. It may take a bit of your time and energy, but you will likely thank yourself later.

> *Instructor should take a moment to express the importance of knowing that you are not alone in your trials, as many prenatal families share similar joys and similar challenges. Because of this, very often, we will share our thoughts and feelings throughout each lesson, and you will have an opportunity to discover what you have in common with others throughout this educational journey. Lets start know! Which Prenatal Care Provider would you like to have? You are welcome to share your reason why as well.*

Places to Deliver Your Baby

- Some women have very strong views about where and how they would like to deliver their babies. There's absolutely nothing wrong with that! Generally, women will choose to deliver at either a hospital, a birthing center, or at home. Lets talk a little more about these options right now.

- Hospitals are a good choice for women with health problems, pregnancy complications, or those who are at risk for problems during labor and delivery. This is because hospitals offer the most advanced medical equipment and doctors that are highly trained in caring for pregnant women and their babies.

- There are a couple of other things to keep in mind when it comes to hospitals. First, a cesarean delivery can be accomplished if it were to become necessary during labor. Second, different types of pain relief options are typically available, including the option of requesting an epidural (a highly effective and common treatment for labor pains).

- Birthing Centers try to provide a "homey" environment for a woman to labor and give birth in. The goal is to make labor and delivery a more intimate and natural process, and one way this is achieved is by doing away with most high-tech equipment and routine procedures that you may normally see in a hospital setting. For example, you may not automatically be hooked up to an IV or have an electronic fetal monitor around your belly the whole time. Instead, a midwife or nurse might check in on your baby periodically using a handheld machine. A special highlight for many women includes the fact that once the baby is born, all exams and care can occur right in front of you (in your room). Obstetricians typically no not deliver babies at birth centers. If you are a healthy woman who is at low risk for problems during pregnancy and low risk for problems during labor and delivery, you may want to consider a delivery at a birth center if you think this would be a good option for you.

- Please keep in mind that (although it's possible that some pain medications may be available) women cannot receive epidurals at a birth center! This is something that you want to be well aware of and comfortable with before choosing a birth center as your desired place for labor and delivery.

- If you want to deliver at a birth center, make sure it has appropriate accreditations, as well as sufficient staffing and supports for breastfeeding endeavors.

- Homebirth is the final option that we will cover today. If you are a perfectly healthy pregnant woman (as far as you and your Healthcare Provider(s) can tell), and you have no risk for complications during pregnancy, labor, or delivery... then perhaps a homebirth can be considered! It is very important to be certain that you have a strong after-care support system in place at home. To many people's surprise, there are some certified nurse midwives and doctors that will deliver babies at home. Keep in mind that many health insurance companies do not cover the cost of care for homebirths, so you will need to get details on coverage from your insurance company if you feel that this would be a good option for you.

- Homebirths can seem scary to some people, but homebirths are actually fairly common, particularly in many countries in Europe. When it comes to the United States, planned homebirths are not supported by the American Congress of Obstetricians and Gynecologists (ACOG). ACOG believes that the safest place to deliver a baby is in a hospital.

- Where and how you deliver your baby is up to you! If you truly feel that a homebirth is best for you, take measures to ensure the safety of you and your baby. For example, you should have a highly trained and experienced midwife along with a very dependable backup plan. Your backup plan should include a readily accessible obstetrician and details on fast and reliable transportation to a nearby hospital (in the event of an emergency).

So, where do you desire to deliver your baby at this point in time? You are welcome to share your reason why as well.

Prenatal Checkups

- During pregnancy, regular checkups are very important. This consistent care can help keep you and your baby healthy. It allows your Healthcare Provider(s) to spot problems (if they occur) and prevent problems during delivery as well. Every woman's case is different, which can cause differences in how often your checkups take place. Typically, routine checkups occur once each month for weeks four through 28, twice a month for weeks 28 through 36, and then weekly for weeks 36 until you give birth to your precious baby (or babies).

- At your first visit you may be asked what seems like an overwhelming amount of questions. Remember that it's important to be honest with your Healthcare Provider(s) so that your team is in a position to help you the best way they possibly can.

Prenatal Tests

- Different tests are used during pregnancy to check and manage your and your baby's health. At your first prenatal visit, your doctor will use tests to check for a number of things, such as anemia, your blood type, and whether dangerous infections are present.

- During the course of your pregnancy, other (more unique) tests may be recommended as well. While some tests are suggested for all women (such as screenings for gestational diabetes and sexually transmitted infections), other tests could be offered based on your distinctive characteristics (which can include your age, personal health history, family health history, ethnic background, results of routine tests, etc.)

High-Risk Pregnancy

- You will need to know whether your pregnancy is considered "high-risk." High-risk pregnancies are those with a greater chance of complications. However, this does not mean there will be problems! It is possible to have a high-risk pregnancy without experiencing complications. So, if you find your pregnancy is high-risk, do not add extra worry! Simply allow your Healthcare Provider(s) to provide a bit of extra care that may be necessary for your case.

- A few factors that may cause your pregnancy to be high-risk include younger age, older age (older than 35 years), overweight status, underweight status, problems in a previous pregnancy, pregnancy with multiples (i.e., twins), or presence of certain health conditions before becoming pregnant (such as HIV, cancer, or high blood pressure). It is also possible to enter a pregnancy low-risk and obtain a high-risk status during the pregnancy. For example, significant health issues could develop during a pregnancy (like gestational diabetes).

- Women with high-risk pregnancies may need prenatal care more often, and sometimes from a specially trained doctor. For example, a maternal-fetal medicine specialist is a medical doctor that cares for high-risk pregnancies. Once again, if your pregnancy is considered high-risk, it does not mean you will absolutely have complications! Make sure to continue enjoying your pregnancy! Also, share any concerns you have with your Healthcare Provider(s) so that they can explain your risks in detail and help you understand any chances of a significant problem.

Prenatal Nutrition

- Nutrition involves eating a balanced diet so that your body gets the nutrients it needs to function and grow properly. According to the American Dietetic Association, women of child-bearing ages should maintain good nutritional status through a lifestyle that optimizes maternal health and reduces the risk of poor growth and development of an unborn baby, and birth defects.

- The key components of a health-promoting lifestyle during pregnancy include appropriate weight gain, appropriate physical activity, consumption of a variety of foods in accordance with the Dietary Guidelines for Americans, appropriate and timely vitamin and mineral supplementation, avoidance of harmful food/drink substances, and safe food handling. This will be covered in Lesson 3.

Nurturing

- Nurturing comes from the Latin word Nutritura. The meaning here is to care for, to bring up, and to nourish.

  To Parent is to nurture (a child). To Live is to nurture (yourself). Ultimately, taking care of yourself will help you to take care of your children, to, because you cannot pour from an empty cup!

- The nurturing of yourself and your (unborn) child should start now (if it has not already started).

Prenatal Nurturing and Nutrition

- So now, lets take a look at the word "prenatal" to understand its role in the phrase Prenatal Nurturing and Nutrition.

- "Pre" means before, and "natal" means born. Therefore, prenatal means "preborn" or, in other words, prior to child birth taking place. The words Prenatal Nurturing & Nutrition are joined to demonstrate that this course is about nourishing yourself and your preborn child (with healthy foods, nurturing care, unconditional love, etc).

Prenatal Nurturing

- There was once a time where many parents thought that they could consider pregnancy as a nine-month grace period before the actual work of parenting begins. Well, those days are long gone! Now, there is plenty of research that shows how lifelong well-being begins in the womb! This includes mental health as well!

Instructor should take a moment to encourage the importance of making good decisions. Example: "Every single thing that you do (even now) will have critical impact and who your child becomes, the types/amounts of opportunities that will present from him or her, and, ultimately, the quality of life they will have! Your current choices are shaping your child's being. Try and set your child up for success by doing the best you possibly can!"

Pregnancy Concerns

- Lets switch gears and talk about Pregnancy Concerns now.

Pregnancy Concerns/Worries

> *Instructor should allow participants to comment on any concerns, worries, or fears that participants (or their partner) might have. Acknowledge each person's comment(s) and thank them for sharing while assuring them that it is likely that other participants here today can relate to what has been shared.*

Common Pregnancy Fears

- Common Pregnancy Fears – If you also have similar concerns as those that were shared, or you have other fears/concerns that weren't mentioned, you are likely not alone. There is a long list of common pregnancy concerns! Here are just a few *(Instructor should pick a few concerns to read out)*:

Water Breaking in Public, Peeing in Pants in Public, Partner or Child's Health, Complications, Preterm Labor, Premature Infant, Eating and Drinking Wrong Things, Too Much Stress, Morning Sickness, Miscarriage, Birth Defect, Laying on Belly, Stretch Marks, Face Appearance Changing, Heavy Lifting, Baby Weight, Sex Never Being the Same, Fading Relationship Love, Jealousy of Baby, Postpartum Depression, Painful Labor and Delivery, Emergency C-Section, Not Getting to Hospital on Time, Embarrassing behaviors during labor, Tearing, Unwanted Interventions, Loss of Privacy, and/or Being a Good Parent.

> *Instructor should offer some comforting words regarding how worries are common and, in most cases, can be overcome. Example: "Rest assured that pregnancy risks are generally low, especially for healthy women, and should not induce a high level of concern."*

General Pregnancy Concerns

• Most concerns fall into one of five categories. The five major categories are concerns regarding the pregnancy itself, uncertainties regarding labor and delivery, concerns about finances, having mixed feelings about being a parent (especially if this is your first child!), and issues surrounding (pregnancy influenced) changes in relationships. Lets tackle these concerns one at a time!

Combatting Concerns about Pregnancy

• We will start with a talk on how to combat concerns about pregnancy. First, make sure you start your prenatal care as soon as possible & attend all appointments.

• Also, attend prenatal classes (such as this one)!

• Don't wait on formal classes for all of your prenatal education. Watch relevant prenatal videos and read relevant prenatal books.

• Remember to communicate well with your Healthcare Provider(s), family/friends, and parents of have already experienced one or more pregnancies.

> *Instructor should encourage participants to share other ways that pregnancy concerns can be combatted. Let them know that they may be helping others (potentially tremendously) with their comments.*

Combatting Concerns About Labor and Delivery

Now, lets talk about how we can combat concerns about labor and delivery.

• Partners (and any other persons who will be active in your labor and delivery) need to know what their roles are. Make sure everyone thoroughly understands and is comfortable with the expectation(s) that you have for them. Be as detailed as possible; you may even want to consider creating a birthing plan!

• Discuss the labor and delivery experience with different experienced parents. Ask them what they anticipated during, what went well, what didn't go as planned, and what may have surprised them.

Instructor should encourage participants to share other ways that labor and delivery concerns can be combatted. Let them know that they may be helping others (potentially tremendously) with their comments.

Combatting Concerns About Parenting

- Now, lets talk about how we can combat concerns about parenting.

- Get registered (as a couple if possible) in a parenting program/course.

- Make sure that you both are constantly working to take an equal role in parenting. No one parent should be overwhelmed; you are in this together!

- Don't be afraid to discuss parenting issues with other parents.

- Educate yourself by watching relevant parenting videos and reading relevant parenting books.

- Talk openly with your partner about concerns, and brainstorm/create plans together regarding how you might combat different issues.

- Ask experienced parents how they adjusted and how they addressed any unique challenges along the way.

Instructor should encourage participants to share other ways that parenting concerns can be combatted. Let them know that they may be helping others (potentially tremendously) with their comments.

Combatting Concerns About Finances

- Now, lets talk about how we can combat concerns about finances.

- Babies are expensive! You may want to have a discussion with your insurance agent to be clear on which expenses are covered and which expenses will be your financial responsibility. You don't want any surprises!

- You could also consider meeting with your banker or financial adviser to set up a financial plan for yourself and for your child's future.

- If money is very tight, you can attempt to discuss different options with your medical team. Hospitals and midwives may be willing to generate payment plans with you for those birth expenses that are not covered by insurance.

- If your income qualifies, you may want to seek out other forms of assistance, such as supportive programs, such as the Women, Infants, and Children (WIC) Program.

> *Instructor should encourage participants to share other ways that financial concerns can be combatted. Let them know that they may be helping others (potentially tremendously) with their comments.*

Combatting Concerns About the Relationship

- Now, lets talk about how we can combat concerns about relationship changes.

- Be ready for a long-term and healthy relationship!

- At your comfort level, communicate about anything and everything! Talk about what you are experiencing and feeling (whether it is good or bad).

- Although this is a miraculous part of your life, and all of the focus may seem to be on your oh so very important unborn baby, don't allow this to make you forget about the other important things in your life! Be sure to continue to nurture your relationship for example. Engage in stimulating conversations, fun outings, and intimate activities that make each other feel heard, important, cared for, and loved.

> *Instructor should encourage participants to share other ways that relationship concerns can be combatted. Let them know that they may be helping others (potentially tremendously) with their comments.*

Pregnancy Wishes

Now, lets talk about our pregnancy wishes!

Prenatal Affirmations

> *Instructor should begin by asking participants to share what an affirmation is to them. Instructor may choose to hear 2-3 responses, time-permitting.*

- Thank you for sharing your thoughts! Lets continue our talk on affirmations.

- New thoughts and feelings of discomfort could consistently pop up throughout your pregnancy. Keep in mind that pregnancy risks are generally low, especially if you are otherwise healthy.

- Also, the same way that worries or concerns can arise, wishes (in the form of hopes and dreams) can arise during this period as well! Lets put more of our energy here! Make sure to honor your wishes! Embrace those thoughts and feelings and work towards manifesting them.

- Simply put, affirmations are healthy, nurturing, and positively empowering statements. One unique thing about affirmations is they are expressed in the present tense as if it already exists or you already have it!

- You can have affirmations specifically for this period of your life, called pregnancy affirmations or prenatal affirmations. Some examples of prenatal affirmations include "I welcome and love the changes in my body" and "My baby hears my laughter."

Prenatal Affirmations - Examples

(Optional) Video: Lets take a look at some more examples of prenatal affirmations by watching a video. While watching, try and pay close attention to which affirmations catch your attention. Take note of the affirmations that resonate well with you. Or, allow these examples to spark ideas for you to create your very own!

> *Instructor should play video: "POSITIVE PREGNANCY AFFIRMATIONS"*
>
> *https://youtu.be/ko2LCrpeC_A?feature=shared*

- There are several benefits of using positive affirmations. Today, I will just mention six of those benefits. One benefit includes the ability to motivate you to act on your wishes and desires! And when you take action, this further boosts your desire to persevere!

- Second, they motivate you to keep your focus where it belongs.. in the goal zone! Goal achievement is helped by keeping your concentration on the end-result that you desire.

- Third, they motivate you to recognize negative thought patterns and transform them into positive ones.

- Fourth, they promote sustainable growth as they influence your subconscious mind to access new beliefs!

- Fifth, they can help to boost your self-confidence, self-concept, and self-esteem.

- Last but not least, self-affirmations have also been shown to decrease (dangerous health-deteriorating) stress!

Fear/Tension/Pain

- Fear, tension, and pain can exist in a vicious cycle. Fear can cause more tension in the body, and more tension can cause more pain, whereas more pain can lead to increased fear. The key is addressing fear... and we can address this by combatting all of our different worries using the methods we discussed today! And also by using prenatal affirmations as another tool to manage fear.

BREAKOUT into Small Groups

Instructor should explain to participants that they will now have the opportunity to discuss a class topic with other prenatal persons in a small-group setting.

- Once you are in your group, reintroduce yourself (by stating your first name and how far along you are in your pregnancy).

- Determine 3 Prenatal Affirmations that are meaningful to you and/or your group. Decide on a spokesperson (a person willing to share on behalf of the group). At the end of your discussions, your spokesperson will be invited to share your group's thoughts with the rest of the class without naming any members of the group. Please be respectful of others' thoughts and opinions, and make sure to never interrupt someone while they are speaking. Most of all, enjoy yourself and embrace this unique opportunity to chat with individuals that are facing similar challenges as you.

Instructor should encourage openness and express the real possibility of gaining new life-long friends through lesson small-group discussions. Once participants have completed their small-group discussions, the instructor should allow spokespersons to share what was discussed. The instructor can invite thoughts and opinions from as many spokespersons as time allows.

Communicate and Connect

- It is very important to communicate and connect with your baby, even now, while your baby is still in the womb. One of the best ways for both partners to begin connecting with their baby is to simply talk to the baby! You should strive to talk to your baby every single day.

- You can absolutely talk to your baby any time you want! However, for anyone that would appreciate some examples (as a starting point), some good times to talk to your baby include during peaceful/quiet moments, during times when you have nurturing thoughts about your baby, moments where you feel the baby's movements, and during times of preparation (such as when you are creating a nursery or purchasing baby items for him/her.

- Some parents feel silly or awkward in simply trying to think of words to say. Communicate with your baby by sharing expectations, hopes, and dreams! You can also ask your baby questions! Some ideas are "How are you okay today?" "Are you sleeping now?" "You surprised me, "You started growing before I even knew you were there!" "What do you look like? Are you a boy or girl?" and "I am super excited about seeing you and holding you in my arms."

- Practice assigning positive attributes to your child as well. You can literally talk to your baby the way you would talk to a young child!

- Make sure that anytime you communicate, it is honest, nurturing, and supportive. Communicating may seem silly at first, but once you figure out what forms and styles of communication work for you and your baby, it'll become easy and fulfilling.

- Communicating with your unborn child is super important because it allows for healthy bonding that helps your baby get to know you better and establishes feelings of security. It also helps you get to know your baby! You may find that your baby responds to you at particular times in unique ways (such as giving mom a kick after she caresses her belly in a playful manner). This bonding enriches both of your lives! It strengthens the divine love that you already have for your baby, and helps you to be more mentally and emotionally prepared to continue a nurturing parent-infant relationship and strongly establish what is only the beginning of great communication with your child.

Connecting to My Baby (Ways to Connect)

- (Optional) Video: There are many ways to communicate and connect with your baby (outside of just talking). Lets take a look at some more examples of different ways we can communicate with our unborn baby.

> *Instructor should play video: "8 Best Ways to Bond with Your Baby in the Womb" https://youtu.be/rA5G7gVDozU?feature=shared*

(video) Connecting to My Baby (Affirmations)

- (Optional) Video: Please know that if this is an area that you struggle with, you can create affirmations specifically for connecting well with your baby. Lets take a look at some examples of this now.

> *Instructor should play video: "Connecting to my Baby in the Womb" https://youtu.be/OkHMwgkGEi4?feature=shared*

Oxytocin

- Oxytocin is a hormone in the body that is released once you have an intimate moment (like a meaningful hug or kiss) or even just an intimate thought. For this reason, it has been nicknamed "the love hormone."

- Remember that each labor contraction is caused by a wave of Oxytocin (the love hormone) coursing through your body. So, very literally, each birthing surge is a surge of love. When the big day arrives, allow yourself to meet each surge with the same warmth, intimacy, and acceptance that you would experience during a kiss or a loving embrace. And in the same way, allow yourself to meet each pregnancy challenge with grace and courage.

> *Instructor should offer some comforting words here. For example, "And remember, these challenges are only temporary (as your pregnancy won't last forever), you and your baby will get through it."*

Connect with your Baby Today

- Make sure to find a way to connect with your baby today.

THANK YOU!

Today's Topics

- Welcome to Lesson 2 of Prenatal Class! Today, we will talk about the changes experienced during pregnancy, basic womb anatomy, pregnancy trimesters, your baby's development in the womb, and the mom's pregnancy development.

> *Instructor should ask participants whether they were able to find a way to communicate with their baby since the last lesson, and invite them to comment on how they accomplished this.*

A Woman's Heart

- "Just as a woman's heart knows how and when to pump, her lungs to inhale, and her hand to pull back from fire, so she knows when and how to give birth." ~ Virginia Di Orio

- In just the same manner, your body knows just what to do for your pregnancy! All your body needs from you is to give it the support that it needs to do the best possible job.

Changes During Pregnancy

- Pregnancy brings about so many changes! Every inch of your being and every inch of your life are surely impacted. From the moment of conception, there are constant spiritual, mental, emotional, spiritual, and even social changes that can and will take place. And lets not forget that these are all connected! So, for example, you may experience physical changes that cause mental changes, mental changes that cause emotional changes, and emotional changes that affect your social life.

- Physical changes tend to be more apparent. Pregnancy brings about distinctive physical changes in the woman's body, especially during the second and third trimesters, and acceptance of all of these changes will be key now.

- Acceptance of these changes can be tough! Particularly if you are a woman whose self-esteem is closely tied to your physical attractiveness, this can be a very challenging time. However, without acceptance of the process, certain pregnancy changes may begin to eat away at your self-worth and could also negatively impact your feelings for the baby. It's very important that you surrender to changes and even embrace these changes. One way to achieve acceptance is through understanding. Once you have a better understanding of why these changes occur and what to likely expect moving forward, you will be in a better position to appreciate the process. We will talk a lot more about common pregnancy experiences today.

SUPPORT

- Guys, I want you to imagine for just a second that one day, as you were minding your business, someone said to you, "Hey! I'm glad you're having a great day! Just wanted to let you know that from this very moment, every aspect of you is going to change. Changes will be constant and, at times, massive and rapid! This will happen for the next 9 months or so, whether you like the changes or not. Good luck!"

> *Instructor should offer comforting words to acknowledge that this is a difficult challenge.*

- Now, ladies, I want you to imagine for just a second that one day, as you were minding your business, someone said to you, "Hey! I'm glad you're having a great day! I just wanted to let you know that from this moment, your partner may have frequent mood swings (seemingly for no apparent reason) and will also become more and more dependent on you for many things. There will be many demands, and you will need to roll with the punches. Also, you will need to totally change your lifestyle to be able to provide any and all supports that are needed in order to help maintain a safe and enjoyable prenatal journey. Good luck

> *Instructor should offer comforting words to acknowledge that there are challenges for guys, too!*

- The bottom line here is that everyone will have their unique challenges, and we need to make sure that we are always doing are best to provide one another with the support needed at any given time. Have grace with one another.

Never Alone

- What if you're thinking, "the 'couples' information doesn't even apply to me?" Completing a pregnancy without your partner can be very challenging, and single-parenting (after the baby is born) comes with unique challenges as well.

- Also, Single-parenting can look different for different people. For example, you could actually be married and still find yourself single-parenting for one reason or another. Keep in mind that you are a great role-model of courage, strength, love, and resilience for your child... you should be celebrated! Re-invent yourself to be an incredible and mighty version of you, a version you never knew was possible!

> *Instructor may add more words of encouragement here.*

- Also, know that you are never 100% alone. Look to family, friends, and different communities that include people who are facing similar challenges as you and can offer you different ideas on how to tackle various obstacles.

Have You Noticed?

Now I would like you to think about any changes you have already noticed. Remember, changes are not just physical! For example, have you noticed changes in sexual activity? Changes in communication between you and your partner? Changes in perceptions of yourself or others? Changes in how your priorities?

> *Instructor should allow participants to share comment on changes they have noticed and thank them for sharing.*

BREAKOUT into small groups

> *Instructor should explain to participants that they will now have the opportunity to discuss a class topic with other prenatal persons in a small-group setting.*

- Once you are in your group, reintroduce yourself (by stating your first name and how far along you are in your pregnancy).

- Discuss what changes you have already noticed (from you and/or your partner). Which category are most of your changes in: physical, mental, spiritual, emotional, or social? Decide on a spokesperson (a person willing to share on behalf of the group). At the end of your discussions, your spokesperson will be invited to share your group's thoughts with the rest of the class without naming any members of the group. Please be respectful of others' thoughts and opinions, and make sure to never interrupt someone while they are speaking. Most of all, enjoy yourself and embrace this unique opportunity to chat with individuals that are facing similar challenges as you.

> *Once participants have completed their small-group discussions, instructor should allow spokespersons to share what was discussed. The instructor can invite thoughts and opinions from as many spokespersons as time allows.*

Physical Changes

- Lets take a close look now at some physical changes that commonly take place during the prenatal period. As we go through these changes, I will also ask about your experience so that you can see what you have in common with others.

- Breasts Enlarge and may even feel very tender. For some women, there is not much change in sensation, while for other women, a simple touch can be very uncomfortable. These changes are in preparation for nourishing the baby. You may experience leaking nipples as well, particularly towards the end of the pregnancy. Changes with breasts are often one of the very first symptoms noticed.

For this section, instructor should ask: Did you or someone you know experience extremely tender breasts? Instructor can take for comments or simply ask participants to acknowledge whether this is True or False.

- Morning sickness is common, especially during the first trimester. It can also happen at any time of the day or night (not just in the morning). If you are struggling with morning sickness, you can try lemon water or ginger products (ginger candies, ginger ale, ginger teas, etc.). Make sure that you are getting enough fluids; staying hydrated is a great way to combat nausea. Also, make sure that you are not hungry! Although eating may be the last thing on your mind during an episode of morning sickness, try getting something down! Even if it means nibbling on some crackers.

- If the nausea does not subside, or you are also experiencing frequent vomiting, tell your Healthcare Provider(s) right away. There are medications available that have been proven safe for pregnant women, which your doctor may offer you.

Instructor should ask: Did you or someone you know experience morning sickness?

- Fatigue can be heavy, but quite frankly, you should be tired! After all, it takes a lot of work to grow a tiny human! Many women find themselves sleeping more and exercising less, and there's nothing wrong with that.

Instructor should ask: Did you or someone you know experience serious fatigue?

- Energy levels can go up and down, and seemingly even left and right, throughout a pregnancy. It is important for expectant mothers to listen carefully to their bodies during this time. If you're thinking you need rest, please rest. If you feel maybe you're thirsty, please get a cup of water. If you feel you need to move your body, get moving! If you feel you need fresh air, please get outside! And so on.

> *Instructor should ask: Did you or someone you know experience fluctuating energy levels?*

- Body temperature is another area of change. If you have been feeling a bit warmer, it's not in your head! Your body temperature is approximately five degrees higher during the prenatal period. This can also cause a bit more perspiration than you are likely used to. If you are struggling with this, you may want to consider investing in a good fan, especially at night (if you are experiencing nighttime sweats). Also, take a closer look at your clothing! You may want to change the type of fabric you wear or change the manner in which you wear layers. You may also find that you are going for more cool drinks, and that is just fine.

> *Instructor should ask: Did you or someone you know experience change in body-temperature?*

- Swelling can occur throughout the body, but particularly with the feet and/or ankles. This is due to fluid retention and can be accompanied with headaches, leg cramps, and even dizzy spells. If you are experiencing extreme swelling, make sure to alert your Healthcare Provider(s) so that they can rule out any potentially serious issues (such as blood clots). You may want to try keeping your legs and feet elevated or putting on a pair of compression socks. Fluid retention can increase as the pregnancy progresses...but don't worry. Typically, swelling begins to decrease as soon as you give birth. Eventually, you will look like your normal, non-puffy self.

> *Instructor should ask: Did you or someone you know experience swelling?*

- Believe it or not, vision change can also occur during pregnancy. These changes can be small or major. However, with any changes to your vision should alert your Healthcare Provider(s) immediately.

> *Instructor should ask: Did you or someone you know experience vision change?*

- Acne can pop up, likely due to the increase of the hormone progesterone. HCG (another hormone) also causes glands to secrete more oil, which could lead to more acne. If you are struggling with this and attempting to tackle it on your own, please be aware that even some topical treatments can be dangerous during pregnancy. Check with your Healthcare Provider(s).

> *Instructor should ask: Did you or someone you know experience acne?*

- Weight Gain is necessary! There is a lot going on! A placenta that is increasing in size, increased blood volume, greater fatty deposits, and, lets not forget… your baby! A sufficient weight gain is 24-35 lbs. Of course, this could be higher or lower, depending on the case.

> *Instructor should ask: Did you or someone you know experience extreme weight gain or even weight loss (during 1st trimester)? Share!*

- Indigestion and heartburn are no fun and can occur because there is a reduction in digestive tract movements, as well as decreased stomach acid. If you are struggling with this, make sure to talk to your Healthcare Provider(s)! Your doctor may suggest certain medications that are safe for you and your baby.

> *Instructor should ask: Did you or someone you know experience indigestion or heartburn?*

- Breathlessness may become an issue and could happen more frequently as the pregnancy progresses. This is due to elevated progesterone. However, this is also due to the fact that you've got a whole entire growing baby in your womb as well.

> *Instructor should ask: Did you or someone you know experience breathlessness?*

- Constipation and urinary problems are also common complaints. The baby pressing down on a woman's rectum, and the intestinal muscles have slowed in function due to pregnancy hormones. Also, if you are taking iron supplements (alone or in <u>prenatal</u> vitamins) for anemia, this can also cause constipation.

- In order to gain some relief, you may want to consider increasing your intake of fibrous foods, drinking more fluids, and exercising. There are also some over-the-counter stool softeners that are helpful and safe to try out. Discuss issues like this with your Healthcare Provider(s).

> *Instructor should ask: Did you or someone you know experience constipation or urinary problems?*

- Stretch Marks are lines on the body (colored pink, purple, dark brown, etc) that appear due to a weakening of elastic tissue of the skin. There is too much stretch without proper hydration for elasticity. For relief, you may want to try belly butter or body oils. Even with this, you should always be working to hydrate from the inside out! Make sure to drink plenty of water every single day.

Instructor should ask: Did you or someone you know experience stretch marks?

Emotional Changes

- Due to the effects of the hormones of pregnancy, there are accompanying emotional changes. Lets look at the hormones first, then we will talk about the associated emotional changes.

- The hormone prolactin causes breasts to grow and make different milk components (like lactose and lipids). This hormone also affects personality and causes women to feel more "maternal."

- Progesterone levels increase throughout pregnancy to help maintain the inner layer of the uterus so it can provide support for your developing baby. This hormone also creates a tranquilizing effect and protects against stress, as well as helps you sleep better!

- Estrogen stimulates the growth of your uterus and improves blood flow between the uterus and the placenta. We will talk more about the placenta in just a moment. Estrogen also prepares your breasts for milk production by enlarging the milk ducts. Estrogen may be associated with changes (both positive and negative) in your mood and sex drive.

- Relaxin does just what you'd think: it relaxes you! More specifically, it relaxes the intrauterine ligaments. Flexibility is super important now, for obvious reasons. This hormone loosens things up a bit (below the belt) in preparation for childbirth. The goal is to ease the baby's passage through the birth canal.

- It relaxes the arteries as well, which is why you are able to handle pregnancy's increased blood volume. On the downside, this hormone does not discriminate! So what happens when the muscle that prevents stomach acid from creeping back into your esophagus becomes floppy? You probably guessed it… heartburn.

- Oxytocin is the feel-good or love hormone that helps us bond with others. During delivery, huge bursts of oxytocin run through the brain. A chemical reaction that happens when a baby's born causes a stimulation of the production of additional oxytocin and intensifies the mother-baby bond.

Moodiness

- A woman's experiences, as well as changes in sleep patterns, eating habits, sex-drive, and energy levels during pregnancy, can all affect her emotional state.

- Also, there are complex biochemical changes taking place every single second, and intense hormonal fluctuations. Certainly, pregnancy is an extremely emotional experience, and there is a lot going on in a woman's head during those 9 months. Sometimes, a pregnant woman's feelings change by the hour! In one instance, there may be feelings of happiness, while in the next moment, feelings of anxiety arise. Hang in there; this is only temporary! Most women find that their moods level out by the middle of pregnancy.

> *Instructor should ask: Did you or someone you know experience moodiness*

Memory Loss

- Have you ever heard terms like "mom brain," "pregnancy brain," or "brain on hold" and wondered whether these were jokes? Well, these are not jokes; memory loss does exist! Women are more forgetful during pregnancy for many reasons, especially in the third trimester." It can be quite frustrating to forget words, appointments, or tasks at times, especially of you are used to being very organized. You may feel like you are going crazy at times… you are not! This is also part of the pregnancy package! But this, too, shall pass.

> *Instructor should ask: Did you or someone you know experience memory loss?*

Vivid Dreams

- Have you been having very bizarre dreams lately? It's actually normal to have extremely vivid and even scary dreams during pregnancy. Many pregnant women report an increase in random, lifelike dreams. This can occur due to spiritual changes or due to hormonal fluctuations, which can make it difficult to differentiate between reality and nightmare. While these dreams seem to heighten in the third trimester, they are normal and typically subside once you give birth to your baby.

> *Instructor should ask: Did you or someone you know experience vivid dreams?*

Identity Crisis

- As a woman's body changes, she may ask herself, "who is this new person?" and experience a bit of an identity crisis. Also, as your dependence on others becomes greater, you may struggle with acceptance of this… especially if you're used to functioning with independence by nature. This could also cause a bit of an identity crisis. Some women experience there "new looks" positively and exude pride in her pregnancy and fertility. The perspective you choose will be up to you.

> *Instructor should ask: Did you or someone you know experience an identity crisis?*

- During the final weeks, the nesting instinct develops, which is characterized by bursts of energy to take preparatory actions for the baby coming! Cleaning the house, preparing the nursery, and having everything ready for the baby. This may be linked to oxytocin. Some women find themselves doing things that they can't fully explain (i.e., cleaning in ways that they have never cleaned before or organizing places that never crossed their mind prior to the pregnancy).

> *Instructor should ask: Did you or someone you know experience nesting? If it was you, what did you find yourself doing?*

Social Changes

- Pregnancy often changes a <u>marriage</u> or a <u>partnership</u>. Changes could be beneficial or not so beneficial. If the relationship was shaky to begin with, and you were thinking that the pregnancy will probably stabilize things, that is not realistic. It is actually a common misperception.

- Ladies, be aware that if you are feeling less attractive, these thoughts will affect your behaviors. Certain behaviors could resemble a subtle distancing, and your partner could interpret this subtle distancing as a rejection. This is another reason why communication is so important now. If communication between partners is weak, such distancing may continue to move partners further and further away from one another.

- **About friends and family**: In a recent poll of 4000 moms, 50% said they lost contact with a group of their friends after becoming pregnant, and 25% said they didn't meet up with any old mates at all.

- If you have lost certain friends (or even family members), it is not necessarily your fault. Insecurity could be a factor. Your baby is a blessing, and someone could be insecure because they're not in the same position as you. This can lead to what appears to be rejection (as they don't want to be reminded that they are on a different path than you, which could cause them to feelings of discomfort, considering they may feel left behind.)

- Find your people! Find those people that are supposed to be with you in this season. The ones who'll be there for you, even when you're not feeling like talking on the phone every day or having a wild night out.

- A study was conducted where 6 in 10 women felt more in tune with other moms going through the same experiences. For many women, meeting a whole new group of women that are also pregnant is a fun and refreshing pregnancy highlight.

Acquaintances and Strangers

- As your pregnancy begins to show, others will (hopefully) begin to extend courtesies that you may not be normally given. This could include things like being given a seat on the bus, getting assistance with carrying/opening packages, having doors held open for you, or being given a "pass" to cut in line to use the bathroom.

Sexual Relationships

- Your sexual desire may go up and down during pregnancy, largely due to changes in hormone levels. But also, changes in the physical characteristics of the sexual organs can affect your desire as well.

- Some women experience a reduced sexual desire towards the end of pregnancy. This could be due to women having a fear of inducing labor.

> *Instructor should ask: Did you or someone you know experience any social changes?*

Physical Approaches

- Make sure that you are always listening to your body. Stretch away tension and learn different relaxation skills (as approved by your doctor). Also, make sure you are getting the sleep that your body needs.

(video) Directed Visualization

- (Optional) Video: Lets do a directed visualization right now! Get nice and cozy, and try to listen carefully. Allow yourself to go "somewhere else" and experience some gentle relief.

> *Instructor should play video: "Female Voice Hypnosis 'The Beach' Guided Imagery Technique"*
> *https://youtu.be/_Vxr3VkKsTY?feature=shared*

- This is just one of many relaxation techniques. If it worked for you, great! If not, you will need to figure out what does work for you. Relaxation activities are super important because they can help us become aware of areas of our bodies where we store tension. These skills will help throughout your pregnancy and can be used whenever you feel stress or tension building. This can also help with the pain and discomfort of labor since we tend to feel less pain when we are relaxed. Also, if you have a support person who has also practiced relaxation exercises, that person can be a greater help during labor and delivery.

> *Instructor should ask: Do you currently have any relaxation techniques that work for you?*

Mental Approaches

- Try adopting a more positive attitude, do things to intentionally increase your self-worth, set realistic expectations, keep a generally positive outlook on life, work on improving your communication skills, leave work at work, and get more organized.

> *Instructor should ask: Do you currently have any mental approaches/techniques that work for you?*

Social Approaches

- Make sure to either find or develop a support network and maintain a social life. Consider volunteer your time to help others. Develop or maintain your sense of humor, and keep up with some special hobbies.

> *Instructor should ask: Do you currently have any social approaches/techniques that work for you?*

Pregnancy and Sleep

- Challenges with obtaining proper sleep are very common during the prenatal period. Pregnancy is associated with many physiological changes that can influence sleep and sleep quality. Many (if not most) pregnant women report a sleep disturbance, such as insomnia. Insomnia can include difficulty initiating sleep, difficulty maintaining sleep, and/or experiencing nonrestorative (not satisfying) sleep. Sleep deficiency is another common complaint, and it involves experiencing a lack of the proper amount of sleep (to note: normal sleep outside pregnancy should be 7 to 9 hours per night).

Sleep is Important, Especially Now!

- Proper sleep is needed for good health! While you're sleeping, very important restorative functions are taking place in the body. Also, women who don't get enough sleep during pregnancy may have higher risks of developing pregnancy complications (such as preeclampsia).

- You may want to invest in more supportive pillows or ask your partner for a back massage on occasion.

(Optional) Video: Lets take a look now at some different methods we can use to get better rest/sleep.

> *Instructor should play video: "2 Common Pregnancy Sleeping Positions Mistakes(& Easy Fixes)"*
> *https://youtu.be/5PNFKQvR550?feature=shared*

> *Instructor should ask participants to share whether they are familiar with any other ways to get better sleep during the prenatal period.*

Anatomy:

Now we will talk briefly about Anatomy.

Taking a Closer Look at the Womb

- Lets talk about some significant parts/features of the womb. Clinically, your baby may be referred to as a blastocyst, embryo, and then a fetus. These are all scientific names for your baby to simply indicate the level of development that they are at. The placenta is extraordinary in that it is a temporary organ that connects your baby to your uterus during pregnancy. The placenta develops shortly after conception and attaches to the wall of your uterus. Your baby is connected to the placenta by the umbilical cord. Together, the placenta and underlined umbilical cord make a powerful team and act as your baby's lifeline while in the uterus.

- The placenta is amazing in its functions! It provides your baby with oxygen and nutrients, removes harmful waste and carbon dioxide from your baby, produces hormones that help your baby grow, passes immunity from you to your baby, and ultimately helps to keep your baby safe.

Embryonic Development

- Now, I will share a few key developmental milestones that your baby is reaching while still in the womb.

- By week 3, major organs such as the brain, spinal, cord, heart, and gastrointestinal tract begin formation. The leg and arm (buds) may even appear!

- By week 5, the heart can begin to beat. The eyes and ears can also be noticeable

- By week 12, sexual differentiation should be complete. In other words, you can find out the gender of your baby with an ultrasound! At some medical institutions, you can now find out the gender of your baby even earlier with a simple blood test.

- By week 16, the baby's movement can be detected by the mother.

- By week 20, eyebrows and hair can be visible.

- By week 28 the nervous system gains a lot of control in its function. The baby's eyes can open and close.

- By weeks 29-32, There is a massive increase in the amount of body-fat, and fingerprints are set.

- By week 37/38, your baby may be considered full-term. However, please keep in mind that many medical institutions now require you to be 39 weeks into your pregnancy before being considered full-term.

- (Optional) Video: Now, lets take a more detailed look at the milestones your baby is reaching. While watching the video, try and pinpoint where your baby is at in his or her process!

> *Instructor should play video: "Fetal Development Week by Week Overview" https://youtu.be/EhUOkTPW7L0?feature=shared*

> *Instructor should comment on how women typically do not know that they are pregnant right away and ask: How far along were you when you found out (for sure) that you were pregnant?*

Mom's Prenatal Development:

- Now lets switch our attention back to mom! We will take a look at what she may be experiencing during this 9-month period. We will begin by looking at pregnancy trimesters. Please keep in mind that everyone's experience is unique. You may hear something that is commonly experienced in the 1st trimester and realize that you did not have that particular experience until the 2nd trimester, or maybe you never have the experience at all! That is fine and normal.

What to Expect in your 1st Trimester [weeks 0-13]

During your 1st trimester, some common experiences/symptoms include: nausea and vomiting, cravings and aversions, heightened sense of smell, and mood swings. This may be a good time to invest in non-scented products!

> *Instructor should ask participants to comment on whether they can relate to these 1st trimester experiences.*

What to Expect in your 2nd Trimester [weeks 14-26] ["Golden Period"]

- During your 2nd trimester, some common experiences/symptoms include round ligament pains, back pain, leg cramps, heart-burn, nipple changes, stretch marks, and feeling the baby move. Round ligament pains can be very uncomfortable; you can talk to your Healthcare Provider(s) about safe options for pain relief.

> *Instructor should ask participants to comment on whether they can relate to these 2nd trimester experiences.*

What to Expect in your 3rd Trimester [weeks 27-40]

- During your 3rd trimester, some common experiences/symptoms include feeling strong kicks and punches from the baby, hemorrhoids, swollen feet, leaking breasts, and frequent urination.

> *Instructor should ask participants to comment on whether they can relate to these 3rd trimester experiences.*

- Please remember to talk to your Healthcare Provider(s) about any type of pain(s) and/or discomfort(s) you may have at any point in time.

- (Optional) Video: Remember, everyone's experience is unique! So lets take a look at personal accounts of what was experienced by different women at different time-points in their pregnancies.

> *Instructor should play video: "Pregnant Women Weeks 7 to 40: What New Symptoms do you Have" https://youtu.be/DNk5UxnmFYI?feature=shared*

- (Optional) Video: Now, lets take a look at one woman's artistic depiction of what a pregnancy could look like over the entire 9-month period.

Instructor should play video: "This is your Pregnancy in 2 Minutes" https://youtu.be/7nw-QA_-ED8?feature=shared

Your Body is Working Very Hard

- You're taking on a lot right now! Pregnancy induces a coordinated response of multiple organs and organ systems, all to support both mom and baby. Your entire body is working very hard every single second for you and your baby! All the changes that are occurring are in efforts to ensure the successful growth and development of the baby while keeping mom safe at the same time. Make sure to take care of your body the way it takes care of you and your baby.

What Happens to Your Organs?

- Ladies, ever wonder how exactly your body makes room for a whole entire baby... plus a placenta!? Certainly, your naturally elastic belly skin creates some space for the baby. However, a fair amount of the extra space is created due to your organs making way for the star of the show! Not only are your organs functioning differently, but they are placed differently, too! Your organs shift as necessary and even squish together to allow space for your uterus to grow and safely house your baby.

- (Optional) Video (play video twice): With this video, we can see exactly what happens with are organs movement during the prenatal period.

Instructor should play video: "Make Room for Baby from You! The Experience" https://youtu.be/yE-l1stWkT4?feature=shared

- So even though you can't see it, the internal changes your body experiences during pregnancy are just as amazing as the external changes (that being the changes that you can see). This occurrence could play a role with certain discomforts, such as breathlessness or difficulties with bladder control.

My Body is Amazing

- Regardless of where you come from, your height, your weight, your ethnic background, or anything else - Your Body is amazing and performing amazing tasks for you and your baby literally every second. Love your body back, and give it the support it needs by taking care of yourself properly. In lesson 3, we will take a look at proper nutrition during this amazing period of your life so that you can provide your body with nutritional support as well.

Show Appreciation for your Baby and your Body Today.

- Make sure to show appreciation for both your baby and your body today.

THANK YOU!

Today's Topics

- We come to Lesson 3 of Prenatal Class! Today, we will talk about dietary needs during pregnancy, challenges with achieving proper nutrition, stress (as it relates to foods), and the potential impact of drugs and & alcohol consumption.

Role as a Mother

- One of the first and most essential ways a woman begins to exercise her role as a mother to her baby is by paying attention to what she eats while she is pregnant. Also, one of the first ways a man can exercise his role as a father is by supporting mom in meeting prenatal nutritional goals!

- Think of it this way - after your baby is born, would you skip your baby's feeding every once in a while just to "take a break" at times? Would you give your baby a snickers candy bar with a cold soda to wash it down? My guess is you would not! And you shouldn't skip a feeding or consume unhealthy things while you are pregnant either.

- Pregnant women tend to have slightly higher diet quality compared to their counterparts who are not pregnant or breastfeeding. However, the intake is still not the best that it can possibly be. For example, many pregnant women do not eat enough fruits, do not eat enough vegetables, do not eat enough dairy, and do not eat enough seafood. Instead, they consume too much sodium, added sugars, and saturated fats, and refined grains.

- Good nutrition is important now, of course, but it is also important before a pregnancy begins, as well as after a pregnancy is over (especially if you plan on breastfeeding).

- To maintain a healthy pregnancy, approximately 200-400 extra calories are needed each day. Extra calories should come from a balanced diet, which we will talk more about today.

- Keep in mind that (depending on your foods of choice) 200-400 calories is not necessarily a whole extra platter of food! You won't need the "eat for two" mentality, but you will absolutely need the "think for two" mentality as you make careful decisions regarding everything that you decide to consume.

Improve Your Diet

- Your diet is very important, especially during pregnancy! You need to get an abundance of nutrients to your baby! If you are thinking to yourself, "my diet is not so great (poor quality), but I have no desire to improve it. I'm okay with having poor eating habits throughout my pregnancy." Then, you should know that there will be an increased risk for miscarriage, increased risk for your baby having poor brain development, increased risk for an abnormally small placenta, increased risk of having a premature or low birth rate baby, increased risk for stillbirth, increased risk for congenital malformations (birth defects), and even increased risk for serious infant illness after the baby is born.

- On the other hand, if you are thinking, "My diet is great (high quality), and I plan on keeping up with it throughout my pregnancy!" or "My diet is not so great, but I'm making a pledge to myself that I'll do my best to improve it." Then, you should know that there will be an increased likelihood for having a healthy, full-term baby, a baby with healthy brain development and greater intelligence, fewer complications during pregnancy, fewer complications during labor and delivery, and easier recovery from labor and delivery as well.

- Remember, no one is perfect, and balance is key. Just make sure to do your very best; that's the most you can do anyway!

> *Instructor should offer a personal example of how they attempt to achieve healthier eating (either now on in the past, prenatal example preferred).*

My Pregnancy Plate

- My Pregnancy Plate is a tool that can be used for healthy eating during the prenatal period. It reflects current science-based information that can be used to get the best possible nutrition throughout your pregnancy.

- During pregnancy, a woman's additional need for micronutrients increases significantly! My Pregnancy Plate shows that a well-balanced pregnancy diet during this period should include an abundance of various (nutrient-packed) plant-based foods. Only moderate amounts of animal-based foods should be eaten. You can use My pregnancy plate to get more information that is more specific to you and your case. However, here are some general guidelines:

- You can consume about 2-3 servings of non-fat, low-sugar yogurt or milk. When you do consume dairy, try and make sure that it is low-fat. Small amounts of healthy fats should also be included in your diet. These (dairy) foods are important because they provide the calcium, riboflavin, protein, vitamin B12, and magnesium.

- You should be taking in large portions of non-starchy vegetables and a variety of whole fruits. It is best (from a nutritional stand-point) to consume these foods in their whole, natural, and organic state (which would not include dried or artificially juiced fruits or veggies). You can consume need about 3-5 servings of <u>vegetables</u> per day, and 2-4 servings of <u>fruit</u>. These foods provide fiber and other nutrients, such as Vitamin A, C, and Folic Acid.

- When it comes to proteins, try to stick with plant-based proteins or lean meats like nuts, beans, chicken, and turkey. If you love your seafood, make sure that you are choosing "low-mercury" options. You can consume 3-4 servings of protein per day. These foods contain niacin, Thiamin, B6 and B12 vitamins, folic acid, magnesium, zinc, and iron (which is a nutrient that promotes healthy blood and a strong immune system).

- You can consume 6-11 servings of whole grains (not refined grains) per day. Try and make a goal for yourself that at least half of the grains are 100% whole grain. This could be applied to foods like bread, oatmeal, brown rice, pasta, or even bagels. Make sure to look for the word "Whole" grain, and check out the ingredients just to make sure!

- You will need to drink mainly water now. You can aim to drink at least 8 glasses of water each day in order to stay hydrated and prevent complications like constipation. Or, a better option includes asking your doctor since he or she can tell you exactly how much water you should be aiming to drink in a single day, based off of your personal health characteristics. Water is super important now. During pregnancy, a woman needs extra fluids in order to feed her increased blood volume and also for amniotic fluid. Also, without enough fluids, the kidneys could become strained, causing them to compensate by retaining fluids.

This information is intended as a guide, and you are encouraged to continue this conversation with your Healthcare Provider(s) (or even your dietician or nutritionist) so that you can be provided with more specific recommendations.

Risky Foods

- Now lets talk about foods you should stay away from! Some foods should be avoided because they can expose an expecting mom and her baby to very dangerous bacteria.

- Stay away from undercooked foods. From meat to eggs and even sprouts, anything that you consume now should be thoroughly cooked. Stay away from unpasteurized drinks as well. This includes milk, juice, and cider.

- Stay away from soft cheeses and cheeses made with unpasteurized milk (due to Listeria bacteria). Sorry, cheese lovers! This includes cheese like feta, brie, and queso, just to name a few.

- Stay away from lunch meats and hot dogs unless you are able to re-cook it to at least 165 degrees Fahrenheit. If you don't own a food thermometer, it may be time to invest in one!

- Stay away from fish that contains high amounts of mercury. This includes fish like shark, king mackerel, and swordfish.

- Lastly, since foods and beverages high in sugar or saturated fat are typically high in calories and low in nutrients, these should be limited.

- Remember, you are not "eating for two," but you are definitely "thinking for two" while you eat!

- Again, this information is only a guide, and you are encouraged to continue this conversation with your Healthcare Provider(s) so that you can be provided with more specific recommendations.

Extra Nutrients Needed During Pregnancy

- You will need lots of extra nutrients to satisfy your baby's needs and your body's (normal and prenatal) needs.

- There are a few nutrients that play a critical role; we will talk about them right now.

- Calcium is a mineral needed for proper bone formation for the baby, but it also increases the mom's bone strength. The need for calcium is most crucial during the months when the fetal bone formation takes place for the baby. Mom, if your diet doesn't supply enough calcium, your baby will surely deplete your supply.

- An iron supplement is typically recommended during pregnancy. This is because it can be difficult to get enough through your diet alone. If you are not already taking an iron supplement, be sure to ask your Healthcare Provider(s) about this! (For example, you may want to ask when you should start and how many milligrams you should be taking daily). The baby accumulates it for early life, and pregnant women need the extra iron to replenish the red blood supply and accommodate the demand created by the increased blood volume.

- Folic Acid is a B vitamin needed for proper cell division, making it very important for a developing baby! It can help to prevent certain birth defects of the brain and spine.

- This is a lot of information, and if you are feeling overwhelmed, that is completely understandable. The best way to make sure that you are meeting your prenatal nutrition requirements is by taking prenatal vitamin supplements. Talk to your Healthcare Provider(s) to determine which prenatal vitamins are best for you. However, keep in mind that taking your prenatal vitamins does not mean you now have a "free pass" to load up on junk food. You will need to continue eating healthy (to the best of your ability), as well.

(Optional) Video: Lets summarize everything we have been talking about by taking a look at this video.

Instructor should play video: "Every Pregnant Woman Should Know | MyPlate for Pregnancy" https://youtu.be/ksQoCFcsByk

Breakout into small groups

Instructor should explain to participants that they will now have the opportunity to discuss a class topic with other prenatal persons in a small-group setting.

- Once you are in your group, reintroduce yourself (by stating your first name and how far along you are in your pregnancy).

- Discuss whether you have been experiencing any pregnancy food cravings or even aversions? If so, what are they? Also, discuss which food(s) or food group(s) that you would like to incorporate into your pregnancy diet more. Decide on a spokesperson (a person willing to share on behalf of the group). At the end of your discussions, your spokesperson will be invited to share your group's thoughts with the rest of the class without naming any members of the group. Please be respectful of others' thoughts and opinions, and make sure to never interrupt someone while they are speaking. Most of all, enjoy yourself and embrace this unique opportunity to chat with individuals that are facing similar challenges as you.

Once participants have completed their small-group discussions, instructor should allow spokespersons to share what was discussed. The instructor can invite thoughts and opinions from as many spokespersons as time allows.

Factors That Can Contribute to Poor Nutrition During Pregnancy

- There are some factors that can make meeting your nutritional goals a bit more challenging. Some of these factors include poverty, work/job, morning sickness, smoking/alcohol, living status, dieting, food quality, weight/ weight gain, previous pregnancy, and stress. We will talk about all of these things, but lets talk a little more about stress right now.

Stress During Pregnancy

- Stress is a normal reaction to any major change in life (such as pregnancy). In some cases, stress can be good. But in other cases, stress can be overwhelming and potentially harmful for both for you and your baby.

Stress-Busting Foods

- There are some foods that can help tame stress in different ways. Comfort foods, like a big bowl of warm oatmeal, can boost levels of calming brain chemical called serotonin. Some other foods can literally cut levels of stress hormones (like cortisol and adrenaline).

- One way that a healthy diet can help counter the impact of stress is by strengthening the immune system and lowering blood pressure.

- The particular foods that can assist in our management of stress tend to be "whole" foods. Lets take a look at a few now!

Complex Carbs

- All carbs can prompt the brain to make more serotonin. However, if you want a steady supply of this feel-good chemical, it's best to eat complex carbs. Good choices include whole-grain breads, pastas, and breakfast cereals, breakfast bars, or even old-fashioned oatmeal. Complex carbs can help with stabilizing blood sugar levels as well.

Simple Carbs

- Dietitians usually recommend steering clear of simple carbs, which do include sweets and soda. However, those pregnancy cravings can be strong! And just a pinch of these foods might provide the satisfaction you desire. They're digested quickly, leading to a spike in serotonin. This "spike" doesn't last long, and there are better options. So, although you might take a pinch every once in a while, make sure that you don't make these a stress-relieving habit. Try your best to limit these foods.

Oranges

- Oranges make the list because of their wealth of vitamin C. Studies suggest this vitamin can curb levels of stress hormones while strengthening the immune system at the same time! In one study of people with high blood pressure, blood pressure and levels of cortisol (a stress hormone) returned to normal more quickly when people took vitamin C before the stressful task.

Spinach

- Without enough magnesium, headaches and fatigue could become an issue. Both of these things can worsen stress. Just one cup of spinach can help you stock back up on magnesium. Don't like spinach? Other green, leafy vegetables are good magnesium sources as well... just find what works for you. Or try some cooked soybeans or a fillet of salmon, also high in magnesium.

Fatty Fish

- To keep stress in check, make naturally fatty fish your new best friend. Omega-3 fatty acids, found in fish like salmon and tuna, can prevent surges in stress hormones and may even help protect against heart disease, depression, and PMS.

Black Tea

- Drinking black tea could help you to recover better from stressful events. One study compared people who drank 4 cups of tea per day (for 6 weeks) to people who consumed a different beverage. The tea drinkers reported feeling more calm and also had lower levels of the stress hormone (cortisol) following stressful events/situations.

Pistachios

- Pistachios, as well as some other nuts and seeds, are good sources of healthy fats. Eating a handful of pistachios (or other nuts like walnuts and almonds) daily could help to lower your cholesterol and protect you against the negative effects of stress. Nuts are rich in calories, however, so make sure to watch your portion size!

Avocados

- One of the best ways to reduce high blood pressure is to get enough potassium. Most people think of bananas when they think of potassium. However, half an avocado has more potassium than a medium-sized banana. A little bit of guacamole, made from avocado, might be a good choice when stress has you craving a high-fat treat. Avocados are high in fat and calories, so make sure to watch your portion size here as well.

Almonds

- Almonds have an abundance of helpful vitamins, such as vitamin E and B vitamins. These vitamins can help you to be more resilient during bouts of stress and depression. To get the benefits, you can snack on a quarter of a cup daily.

Raw Vegetables

- Crunchy raw vegetables can help ease stress in a unique way… that being a purely mechanical way. Munching on raw veggies (such as celery or carrot sticks) helps to release a clenched jaw, and that can ward off tension.

Bedtime Snack

- Carbs at bedtime can speed up the release of serotonin, which can actually help you to sleep better. However, heavy meals before bedtime can trigger heartburn. Because of this, you will want to make sure to stick to something light (like fruit or low-fat yogurt).

Milk

- Another bedtime stress buster is a tall glass of warm milk. Research shows that calcium eases anxiety and mood swings linked to PMS. Dietitians typically recommend skim or low-fat milk. You can also try plant-based milks that are higher in calcium.

Herbal Supplements

- There are many herbal supplements that potentially fight stress. One of the best studied is St. John's wort, which has shown benefits for people with mild to moderate depression. Although more research is needed, the herb also appears to reduce symptoms of anxiety and PMS. Valerian root is another herb found to have a calming effect. Tell your Healthcare

Provider(s) about any supplements you take so they can check on any possible interactions and make sure that it's safe for you and your baby.

MORE ROADBLOCKS TO PROPER PRENATAL NUTRITION

- We mentioned several roadblocks to proper nutrition earlier. Lets talk about them in a little more depth now. It's good to have a strong awareness of your challenges; that way, you know what to watch for and what to work on moving forward.

Working

- Having a job during pregnancy may contribute to increased stress. With increased stress, there may be a greater likelihood of increased fatigue. With high stress and fatigue, neglect (regarding proper nutrition) becomes likely.

Severe Morning Sickness

- Morning sickness can lead to reduced intake of food and water in general. This inevitably means that there is a diminished amount of nutrients consumed, as well as an increased risk of dehydration.

Other Factors

- Here are some other factors to keep in mind.

- If you eat out frequently, be aware that restaurant-bought food tends to have lots of what we don't need and little of what we do need. These foods are typically high in fat and calories while low in protein and other needed nutrients.

- Very low weight gain could be related to an inadequate intake of protein and calories needed for a baby's growth.

- If you came into the pregnancy with a very low weight or a very high weight, this could indicate poor dietary habits in general. It may be time to take a closer look at your personal eating habits.

- If you were recently pregnant (meaning you were pregnant within a year from your current pregnancy), you may have lowered stores of very important nutrients in your body, such as iron. This could lower the body's defense systems.

Other Factors (cont.)

- Living alone could be problematic because no one is watching! You behave differently when there is someone else around, even if you don't realize it. With little to no accountability, women may not feel as motivated to consistently prepare balanced, healthy meals.

- Dieting can cause you to miss out on much-needed protein, as well as other nutrients, which can be very dangerous for your baby's development of vital organs and body tissues. Also, a lack of calories and nutrients can cause intrauterine growth or retardation for the baby.

- A vegetarian diet is not a bad thing, but it does need to be carefully planned in order to achieve a balanced intake of all necessary nutrients.

Prenatal Exercise

- Have you ever asked yourself whether or not exercising while pregnant is a good idea? Well, the answer is yes! In fact, it's a very good idea!

- Regular exercise during pregnancy can offer you many benefits like shorter and less complicated labor, less need for medical intervention, more energy during pregnancy, faster recovery after giving birth, faster return to their pre-pregnancy weight, and a decrease in various discomforts of pregnancy.

- Keep in mind that your exercise routine does not have to be strenuous. A simple 20-30 minute walk 3-5 days out the week could be just fine. If you were not working out prior to your pregnancy, now is NOT the time to take on elaborate workout routines. Also, even if you were the greatest athlete in the world prior to your pregnancy, you'll still need to adjust your routines as your pregnancy progresses to accommodate your changing body.

- Please remember that your exercise plans should be discussed with your doctor.

Q & A – Smoking/Alcohol/Medication

- Lets go over some myths and facts relating to drugs and alcohol use during Pregnancy. I will read a few different statements, and I want you to respond with whether you think the statement is true or false. Lets get started!

- Smoking during pregnancy is not detrimental to the baby's health.

- **The answer? FALSE.** Smoking during pregnancy is absolutely detrimental to a baby's growth and health. Even second-hand smoke is detrimental (to the health of everyone, baby included). Pregnant women should stay clear of smoke in any capacity (including smoke-filled rooms and close contact with people who smoke). Nicotine decreases the blood supply to the placenta and, therefore, to the baby. Also, diminished fetal development and retarded brain growth increase in proportion to the number of cigarettes smoked each day.

- Taking prescription drugs during pregnancy is okay.

- **The answer is TRUE and FALSE!** Taking prescription drugs during pregnancy is potentially harmful if taken without the supervision of a physician. Your Healthcare Provider(s) should be aware of any prescription drugs you are currently taking (immediately) so that they can make sure that it is safe for pregnancy.

- Cats and birds should be avoided when pregnant.

- **The answer is TRUE.** Cats (particularly outdoor cats and kitty litter) and birds may carry diseases that could make an unborn baby become ill.

- Drinking coffee while pregnant has no harmful effects on an unborn baby.

- **The answer is FALSE.** Caffeine should be eliminated or significantly reduced (to less than 200mg per day) during pregnancy. Some food products that can be very high in caffeine include coffee, cola, tea, and chocolate.

- Taking small amounts of marijuana once in a while won't harm an unborn baby.

- **The answer is FALSE.** When a pregnant woman takes a drug, so does the baby. Also, the baby is still developing and has limited capabilities to get rid of the drug from his/her system.

- Addictive drugs (like heroin, crack, crack cocaine, and marijuana) should never be used when pregnant.

- Keep in mind that today's marijuana is more potent than it was in the past. Prenatal use of marijuana has been associated with infertility, placental complications, and fetal growth retardation. Long-term effects (of the prenatal use of marijuana) on the unborn child include poorer executive functioning skills, increased conduct and behavior problems, poorer school achievement, hyperactivity, impulsivity, and inattention. Some potential immediate effects on the baby include increased startles and tremors and altered sleep patterns (including a decrease in quiet sleep and increased sleep motility).

- It's ok to eat fresh tuna while you are pregnant.

- **The answer is FALSE.** Small quantities of canned tuna is okay. But make sure to avoid freshwater fish while you are pregnant since they are more likely to be contaminated with pesticides and carcinogens.

It's okay to gain about 25 pounds during pregnancy.

- **The answer is TRUE.** A sufficient weight gain is 24-35 lbs. However, if you entered your pregnancy with an underweight status, you may need to gain a bit more (at least 28-40 lbs.), and if you entered your pregnancy with extra weight, your Healthcare Provider(s) may ask you to gain a bit less (approx. 10-25 pounds).

- Only about 2-4 pounds come on during the first trimester. The remainder is added at a rate of about ¾ to 1 pound per week. You may find that you lose weight during the 1st trimester due to morning sickness. By nature's design, when the nausea from the 1st trimester has calmed down, you will catch up with your weight gain just fine.

- Drinking alcohol while pregnant can cause fetal alcohol syndrome.

- **The answer is TRUE.** Drinking wine, beer, and hard liquor during pregnancy has been found to cause a condition known as Fetal Alcohol Syndrome.

- There is no safe amount or safe type of alcohol to consume during pregnancy. Any amount of alcohol, even one glass of wine, passes from the mother to the baby. Also, a developing baby can't process alcohol, so they absorb all the alcohol and have the same blood alcohol content as the mom does.

- Alcohol causes more harm than heroin or cocaine during pregnancy. The Institute of Medicine says, "Of all the substances of abuse, alcohol produces by far the most serious neurobehavioral effects in the fetus."

- Pregnant women who drink run the risk of causing fetal abnormalities ranging from diminished fetal growth to unusual facial features and mental retardation. In fact, alcohol consumption during pregnancy is the leading preventable cause of Mental Retardation. Say no to alcohol during the prenatal period.

Smoking & Alcohol Use

- Now, lets do a quick recap.

- Smoking reduces mom and baby's ability to make use of important nutrients, like vitamin A and vitamin C.

- Smoking also retards taste buds and decreases appetite.

- Alcohol use contributes to poor nutrition for the mom and decreased ability for baby to use nutrients. Also, mom is gaining empty calories.

How Do I Quit Smoking

- If you are a smoker and are interested in quitting, there are some resources that can provide you with some support for this.

> *Instructor should speak on local support resources.*

54

- To give an example: Baby and Me Tobacco Free is a Virtual Program for pregnant women at less than 36 weeks and current tobacco users. There is no age limit, no income or insurance restrictions. There are a total of 10 sessions (some happening pre-delivery and some happening post-delivery), and you can earn vouchers for diapers and wipes!

Help for Drug Abuse or Alcoholism

- If you consume alcohol and are interested in stopping, talk to your doctor, who may be able to assist in getting any necessary treatments. Also, there are some more resources that can provide you with some support for this.

> *Instructor should speak on local support resources.*

Key Takeaways

- (Optional) Video We have covered a lot of information in these classes (from self-care to nutrition to proper sleep and so on). So, lets recap now with some key takeaways.

> *Instructor should play video: "Planning for a Baby: 6 Tips" https://www.youtubeeducation.com/watch?v=epIg4LsYSh8*

Embrace the Journey

- This is an amazing and exciting period for you and your baby--Make sure to embrace every second of this journey!

> *Instructor should offer strong words of encouragement and wish participants well on their pregnancy journey.*

Thank you.

Prenatal Nurturing & Nutrition - Session 1

PNN Lesson1 Worksheet

1. Please provide 1 or 2 reasons why bonding between a parent and their unborn baby is important. *

_____

_____

2. Please provide 1 or 2 reasons why Prenatal Care is important.   *

_____

_____

3. Please provide 1 or 2 situations that may cause a person to be in the "high-risk" pregnancy category. *

_____

_____

4. Please provide 1 or 2 ways that you can communicate with your baby. *

_____

_____

Prenatal Nurturing & Nutrition - Session 2

PNN Lesson2 Worksheet

1. Please provide 1 or 2 ways that hormonal changes can affect you, emotionally. *

   _____

   _____

2. Please discuss a relaxation technique that may work for you. *

   _____

   _____

3. Please discuss 1 or 2 methods you can try in an effort to increase the quality
   of your sleep. *

   _____

   _____

4. Please descr be 1 or 2 first, second and/or third trimester symptoms that should be
   shared with a medical doctor when/if experiencing. *

   _____

   _____

Prenatal Nurturing & Nutrition - Session 3

PNN Lesson3 Worksheet

1. Please discuss 1 or 2 ways that the use/consumption of alcohol or tobacco products can affect an unborn baby? *

   _____

   _____

2. Please provide 1 or 2 benefits of exercising during pregnancy. *

   _____

   _____

3. Please name 1 or 2 foods that should be avoided during pregnancy. *

   _____

   _____

4. Please discuss 1 or 2 foods/food-groups that are important to consume during pregnancy. *

   _____

   _____

Prenatal Nurturing and Nutrition Post-Test

Prenatal Nurturing and Nutrition Exam

PNN Lessons 1-3 Post Test

1) The hormone responsible for bonding between mom and baby and is often called the "LOVE" hormone is Oxytocin.
   a) True
   b) False

2) Most emotional changes during pregnancy are caused by the effects of hormonal changes.
   a) True
   b) False

3) Relaxation activities may help us become aware of areas of our bodies where we store tension.
   a) True
   b) False

4) Sleep related difficulties are not common for a pregnant woman.
   a) True
   b) False

5) Swollen feet, frequent urination, strong movements from the baby are a few common experiences during the first trimester.
   a) True
   b) False

6) Prenatal care should begin as soon as a woman suspects or knows that she is pregnant.
   a) True
   b) False

7) High-risk pregnancies are those with a lower chance of complications.
   a) True
   b) False

8) I should communicate and connect with my unborn child on a daily basis.
   a) True
   b) False

9) The use/consumption of tobacco and alcohol in small amounts is okay during pregnancy.
   a) True
   b) False

10) Some benefits for exercising during pregnancy (as permitted by your doctor) include more energy during pregnancy, a decrease in the common discomforts of pregnancy, and a faster recovery after birth.
   a) True
   b) False

11) A poor quality diet increases the risk of suboptimal fetal development.
   a) True
   b) False

12) My Pregnancy Plate is a tool that can be used for healthy eating during the prenatal period.
   a) True
   b) False

Prenatal Nurturing and Nutrition Exam Answer Key:

1. T

2. T

3. T

4. F

5. F

6. T

7. F

8. T

9. F

10. T

11. T

12. T

References

1. Bavolek, J. D., & Naki, B. (2008). Nurturing Program for Prenatal Families. Family Resources, Inc. Retrieved from www.nurturingparenting.com

2. Johns Hopkins Medicine. (2023). Staying Healthy During Pregnancy: Get a Good Night's Sleep. Retrieved from https://www.hopkinsmedicine.org/health/conditions-and-diseases/staying-healthy-during-pregnancy/get-a-good-nights-sleep-during-pregnancy#:~:text=Lack%20of%20sleep%20is%20more,Gestational%20diabetes

3. Centers for Disease Control and Prevention. (n.d.). Pregnancy Weight Gain Tracker. Retrieved from https://www.cdc.gov/reproductivehealth/pdfs/maternal-infant-health/pregnancy-weight-gain/tracker/single/overweight_tracker_508tagged.pdf

4. Oregon Health and Science University. My Pregnancy Plate (2015).

5. FoodSafety.gov. (2023). Food Safety for Pregnant Women. Retrieved from https://www.foodsafety.gov/people-at-risk/pregnant-women

6. Pincuary, M., & Teubert, D. (2010). Effects of parenting education with expectant and new parents: A meta-analysis. Journal of Family Psychology, 24(3), 316-327. https://doi.org/10.1037/a0019691

7. Parents.com. (2023). Top Pregnancy Fears You Can Feel Better About. Retrieved from https://www.parents.com/pregnancy/my-life/top-pregnancy-fears-you-can-feel-better-about/

8. Customized Inc. (2016). The Importance of Affirmations During Pregnancy. Retrieved from https://www.customizedinc.com/blog/january-2016/the-importance-of-affirmations-during-pregnancy#:~:text=Simply%20put%2C%20affirmations%20are%20short,My%20pregnant%20body%20is%20beautiful.%E2%80%9D

9. National Institute of Child Health and Human Development. (2021). Before Birth. Retrieved from https://www.nichd.nih.gov/health/topics/infantcare/conditioninfo/before-birth#

10. World Health Organization. (2023). Nurturing Care. Retrieved from https://www.who.int/teams/maternal-newborn-child-adolescent-health-and-ageing/child-health/nurturing-care

11. Daelmans et al. (2021). Nurturing Care for Early Childhood Development: Global Perspective and Guidance. Indian Pediatrics. 1: S11-S15.

12. Johns Hopkins Medicine. (2023). Nutrition During Pregnancy. Retrieved from https://www.hopkinsmedicine.org/health/wellness-and-prevention/nutrition-during-pregnancy

13. MedlinePlus. (2021). Pregnancy and Nutrition. Retrieved from https://medlineplus.gov/pregnancyandnutrition.html

14. Ecklund, E. H., & Karney, B. R. (2019). Doulas and Birth Outcomes: A Systematic Review and Meta-Analysis. Journal of Marriage and Family, 81(2), 384–404. https://doi.org/10.1111/jomf.12566

15. Ecklund, E. H., & Karney, B. R. (2020). Doula Care Across the Maternity Care Continuum and Impact on Maternal Health: Evaluation of Doula Programs Across Three States Using Propensity Score Matching. Retrieved from https://www.ncbi.nlm.nih.gov/pmc/articles/PMC7564610/

16. Healthline. (2020). Pregnancy Trimesters: Everything You Need to Know. Retrieved from https://www.healthline.com/health/pregnancy/calendar

17. Google Stock Photos (2023). [Series of prenatal-related images for classroom purposes]

18. Nwadike, V.R. (2021) Pregnancy Trimesters: A Guide. Medical News Today. https://www.medicalnewstoday.com/articles/323742

19. Sherman D.K., Cohen G.L., Nelson L.D., Nussbaum A.D., Bunyan D.P., Garcia J. (2009). Affirmed yet unaware: exploring the role of awareness in the process of self-affirmation. Journal of Personality and Social Psychology, 97(5), 745.

20. Critcher C.R., Dunning, D. (2014). Self-Affirmations Provide a Broader Perspective on Self-Threat. Society for Personality and Social Psychology. Volume 41, Issue 1.

Prenatal Nurturing & Nutrition

session1

Madonna Igah-Okoro, Ph.D, M.P.H., B.S.

MEET YOUR EDUCATOR

- Passion: **XXXXXXX**
- Background: **XXXXXXX**
- Contact Information:

  phone: **XXXXXX**

  email: **XXXXXXX**

Please insert image of

Course Instructor:

XXXXX

XXXXXXX

Introductions

1. My name is ...

1. I am expecting my child on ...
   - This is my first pregnancy.
   - This is not my first pregnancy ...

3. Something unique about me is ...

What You'll Learn

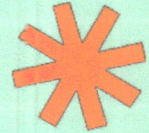

Evidence Based Curriculum

Prenatal Nurturing skills, tips and strategies!

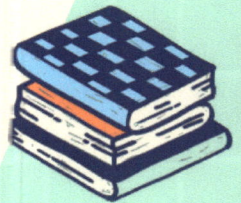

It's my hope that throughout the completion of this course you grow in confidence and skills to live and cultivate a Nurturing Pregnancy!

Course Topics Covered:

LESSON 1:
- Prenatal Nurturing & Nutrition (Meaning)
- Pregnancy Concerns & Pregnancy Wishes

LESSON 2:
- Physical, Emotional, Social, Mental, and Spiritual Changes.
- Mom and Baby's Prenatal Development

LESSON 3:
- Prenatal Nutrition
- Prenatal Substance Use/Abuse

6 Golden Reminders

For a fun and productive class!

1. **Be Visible** (if joining virtually)

2. **Be On Time**

3. **Be Open Minded & Non-Judgmental**

4. **Be an Active Participant**

5. **Be Committed and Connected**

6. **Be Respectful & Maintain Confidentiality**

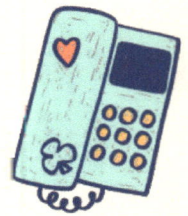

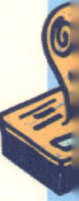

Class Information:

Class Start Date: XXXXX
Class End Date: XXXXX
Day of the Week: XXXXX
Time: XXXXX
Virtual Link (if applicable): XXXXX

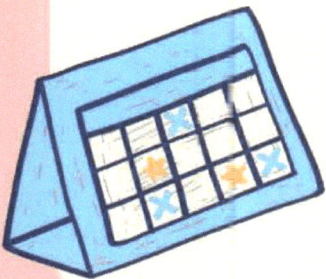

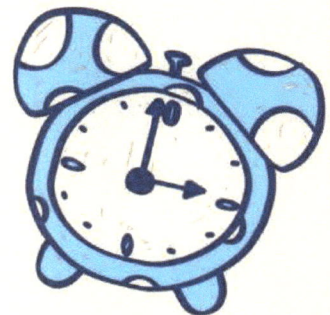

Today's Lesson Topics:

- **Discussion on Prenatal Care.**

- **Defining: Prenatal, Nurturing, and (Prenatal) Nutrition.**

- **Pregnancy Hopes and Wishes.**

- **Pregnancy Concerns and Fears.**

- **Connecting with Unborn Baby.**

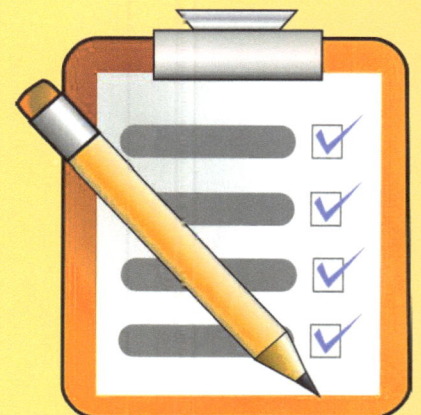

Prenatal Care

- The health care a woman gets during pregnancy is called Prenatal Care.

- Prenatal care should begin as soon as possible!

- Early and regular prenatal visits are very important.

Prenatal Care (cont.)

A Few Things to Keep in Mind!

1. Choosing a Prenatal Care Provider
2. Places to Deliver Your Baby
3. Prenatal Checkups
4. Prenatal Tests
5. High-Risk Pregnancy
6. Prenatal Nutrition

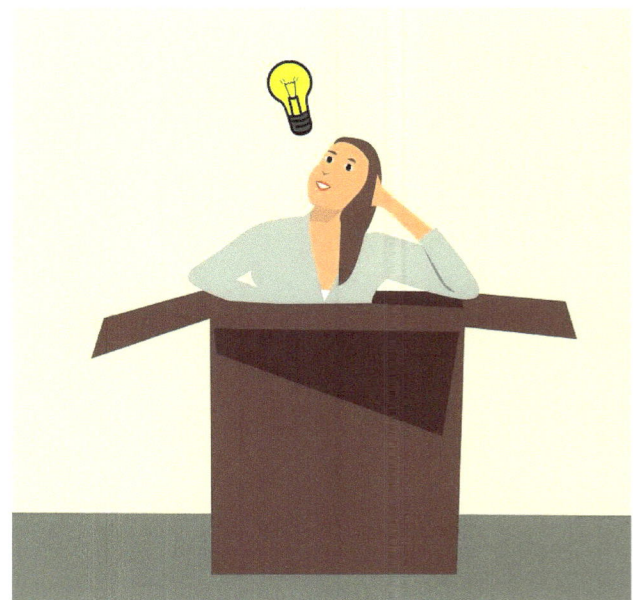

Choosing a Prenatal Care Provider

Obstetrician

Medical Doctors who specialize in the care of women and their unique issues.

Family Practice Doctor

Medical doctors who provide care for the whole family.

Certified Midwife

Provide pregnancy, delivery, and postpartum care.

Doula

Professional labor coach.

★ **ask around for important provider recommendations!**

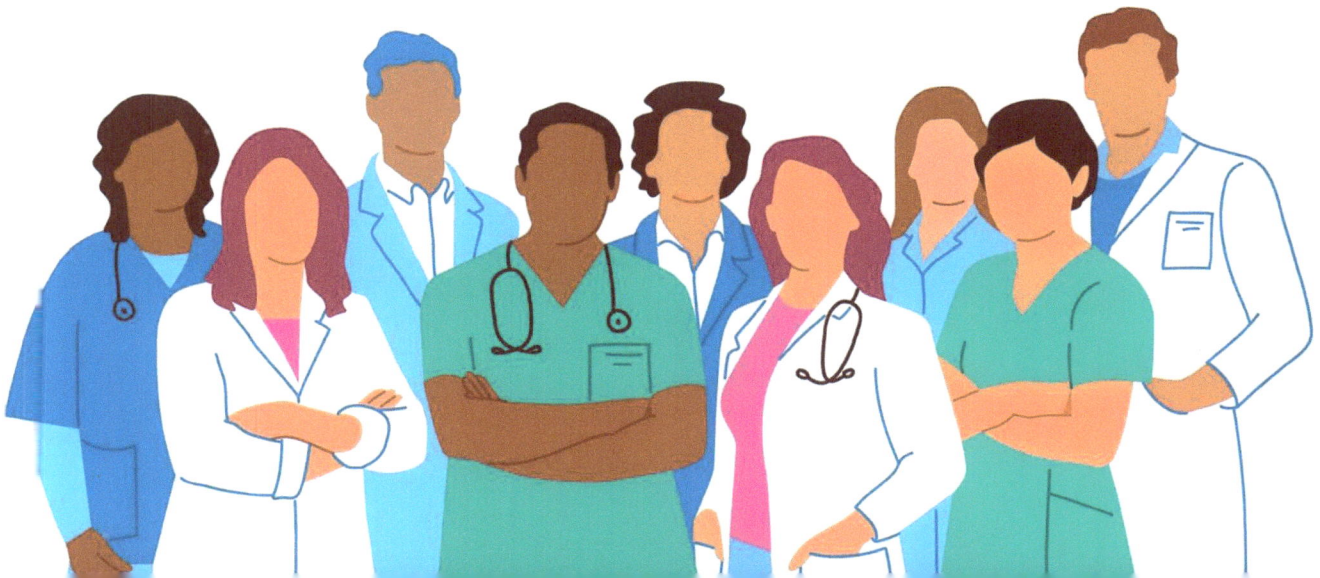

Places to Deliver Your Baby

Hospital
Persons who are at risk for problems during labor and delivery.

Birthing Center
Provide a "homey" environment for labor and delivery.

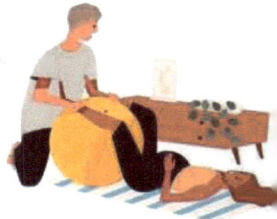

Home (homebirth)
Persons who are not at risk for problems during labor and delivery.

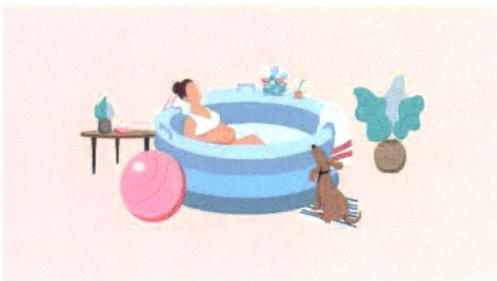

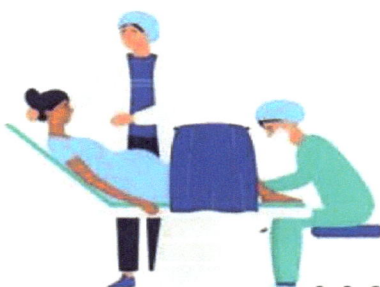

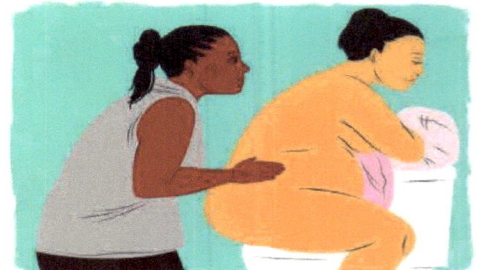

Prenatal Checkups

Routine Checkups:

- Once a month for weeks 4 through 28

- Twice a month for weeks 28-36

- Weekly for weeks 36-40+

Prenatal Tests

- **Different Tests will be Used Throughout Pregnancy in order to Check Mom and Baby's Health Status.**

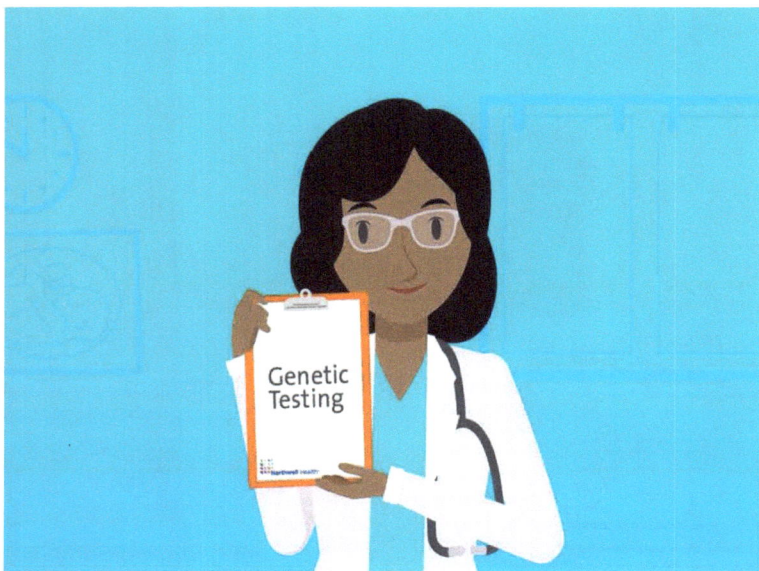

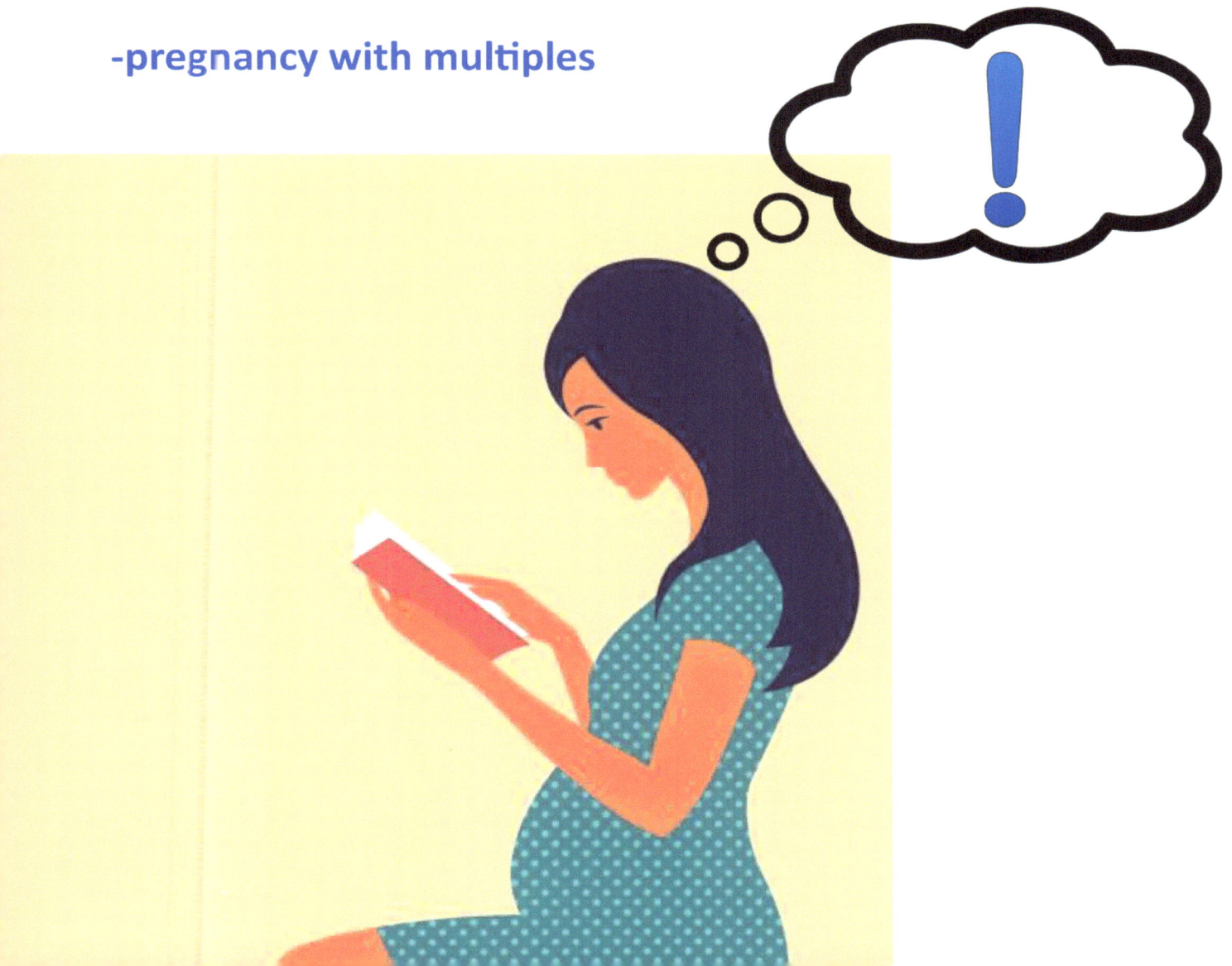

High-Risk Pregnancy

-younger/older

-underweight/overweight

-problematic previous pregnancy

-existing health condition(s)

-pregnancy with multiples

Prenatal Nutrition

- Nutrition is about eating a healthy and balanced diet so your body gets the nutrients that it needs to function and grow.

  -During pregnancy, nutrition is extremely important.

The Academy of Nutrition and Dietetics recommends:

- **Appropriate weight gain**
- **A balanced diet**
- **Regular exercise**
- **Appropriate and timely vitamin and mineral supplementation.**

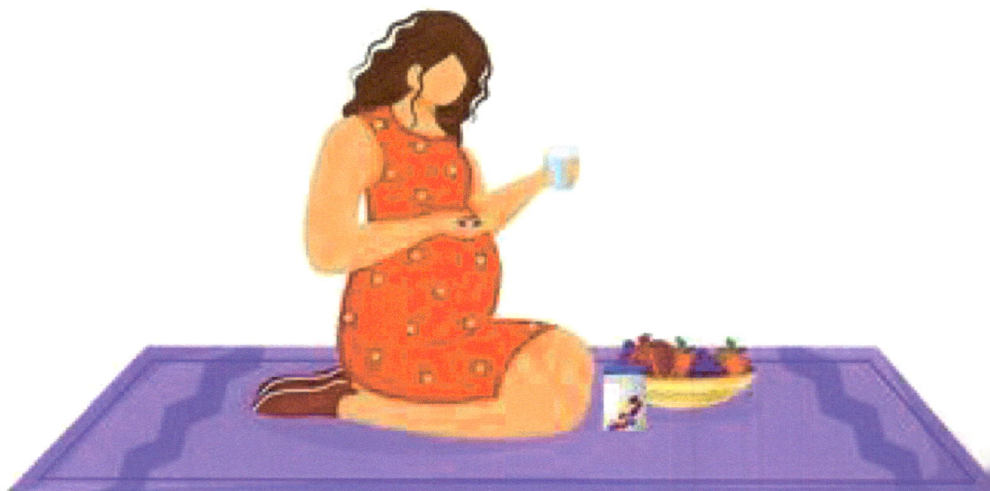

Nurturing

- Nurturing comes from the Latin word Nu tri tura which means to care for, to bring up and to nourish.

  - To parent is to nurture (a child).
  - To Live is to nurture (yourself).
  - Nurturing yourself helps you to nurture your child's self.

Prenatal Nurturing & Nutrition

❖ **PRE** means before

❖ **NATAL** means born

❖ **PRENATAL** means preborn

❖ **NUTRITION** is defined as "the process of taking in food and converting it into energy and other vital nutrients required for the maintenance of life."

❖ **NURTURING** comes from the Latin word Nu tri tura which means to care for, to bring up and to nourish.

❖ **PRENATAL NURTURING & NUTRITION** is all about nourishing our preborn child with proper love, care, and the nutrients necessary for proper growth and development.

Prenatal Nurturing

Science has shown the critical importance of the early years, **starting from pregnancy**, for early childhood development.

PREGNANCY CONCERNS

Pregnancy Concerns/Worries

- Respond to the following statement(s) as it relates to your circumstances:

  - One issue that seems to be a concern for me regarding the pregnancy is...

  - One issue my partner has mentioned that seems to be a concern to him/her regarding the pregnancy is...

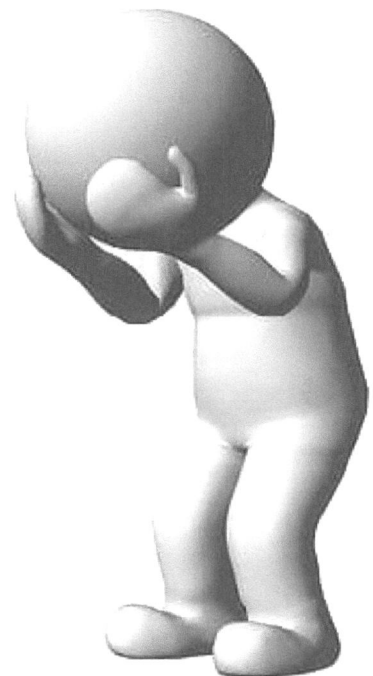

Common Pregnancy Fears & Concerns

1. Water Breaking in Public
2. Peeing in Pants in Public
3. Partner or Child's Health
4. Complications (ie Preeclampsia)
5. Preterm Labor
6. Premature Infant
7. Eating and Drinking Wrong Things
8. Too Much Stress
9. Morning Sickness
10. Miscarriage
11. Birth Defect
12. Laying on Belly
13. Stretch Marks
14. Face Appearance Changing
15. Heavy Lifting
16. Baby Weight
17. Sex Never Being the Same
18. Fading Relationship Love
19. Jealousy of Baby
20. Postpartum Depression
21. Painful Labor and Delivery
22. Emergency C-Section
23. Not Getting to Hospital on Time
24. Embarrassing behaviors during labor
25. Tearing
26. Unwanted Interventions
27. Loss of Privacy
28. Being a Good Parent

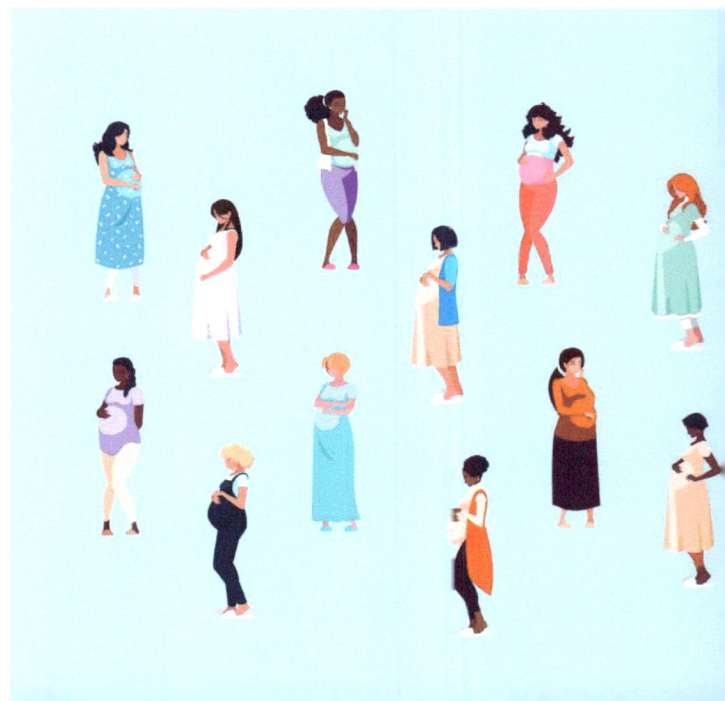

General Pregnancy Concerns

1. Pregnancy Uncertainties.

1. Labor and Delivery Uncertainties.

1. Financial Uncertainties.

1. Parenting Uncertainties.

5. Relationship Uncertainties

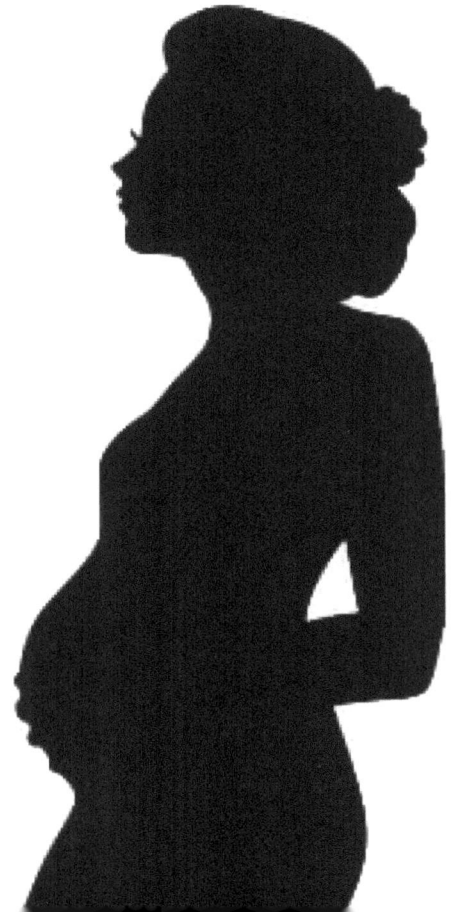

Combatting Concerns About Pregnancy

- ✓ Get Involved Early
- ✓ Learn as Much as You Can
- ✓ Attend Prenatal Appointments
- ✓ Watch videos, Read books
- ✓ Keep Communicating
- ✓ Talk to Your Physician
- ✓ Talk to Others

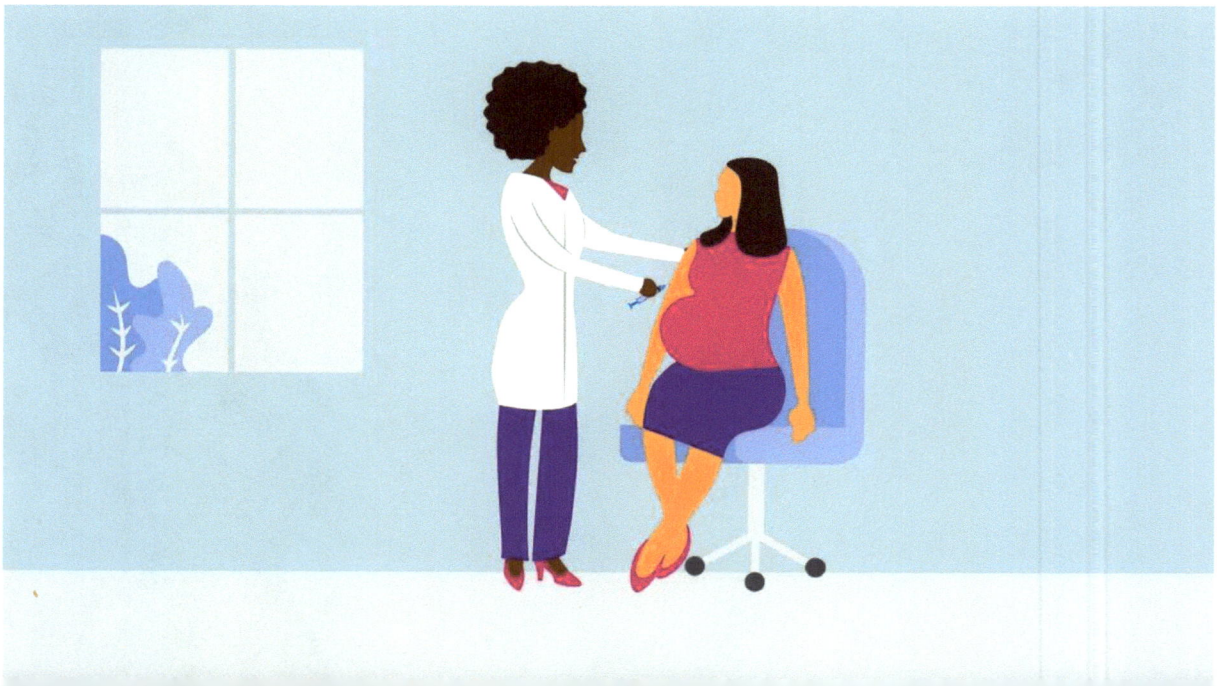

Combatting Concerns About Labor and Delivery

✓ Establish Family
  Member's Roles

✓ Discuss the Details

✓ Make a Birthing Plan

✓ Attend ChildBirth
  Classes

✓ Discuss with other
  Parents

Combatting Parenting Concerns

✓ Attend a Parenting Class

✓ Make sure Parenting Roles are Equal

✓ Discuss with other Parents

✓ Consider Infant Massage

✓ Watch videos & Read Books.

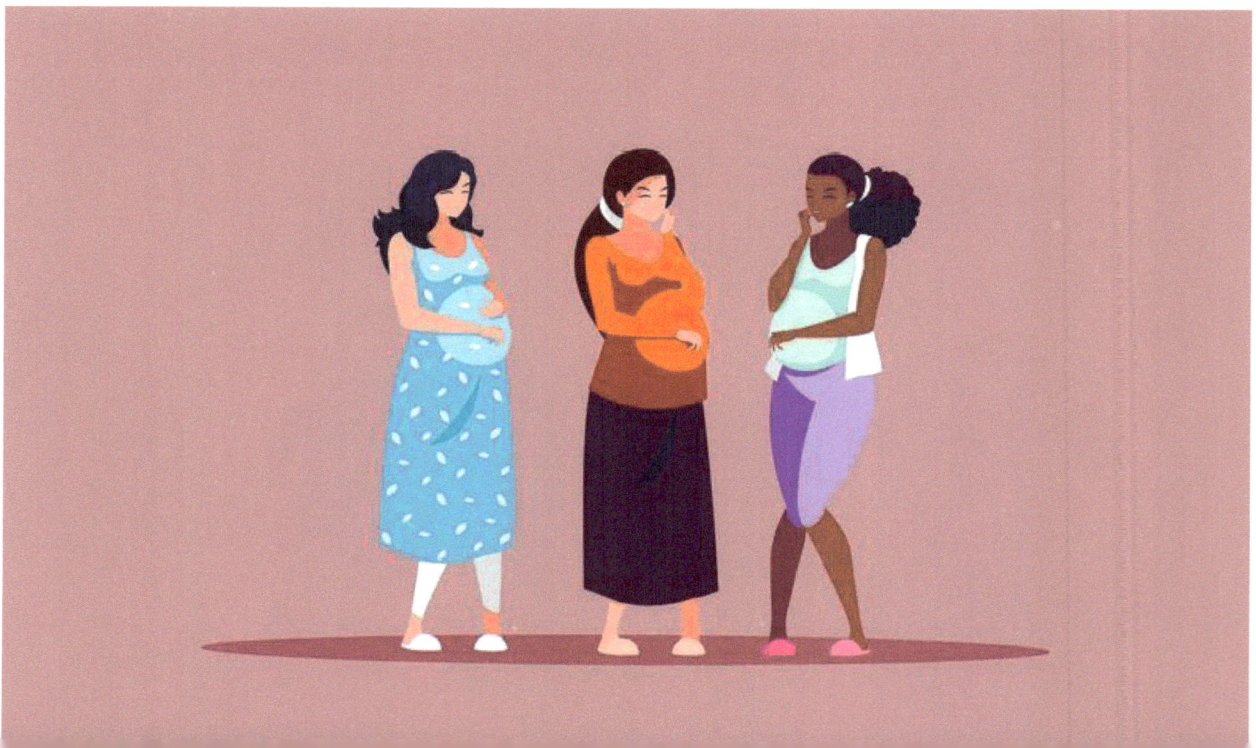

Combatting Concerns About Finances

✓ Get familiar with your insurance agency

✓ Meet with a Banker or Financial Planner

✓ Discuss Payment Plans with your Hospital

✓ Consider obtaining assistance

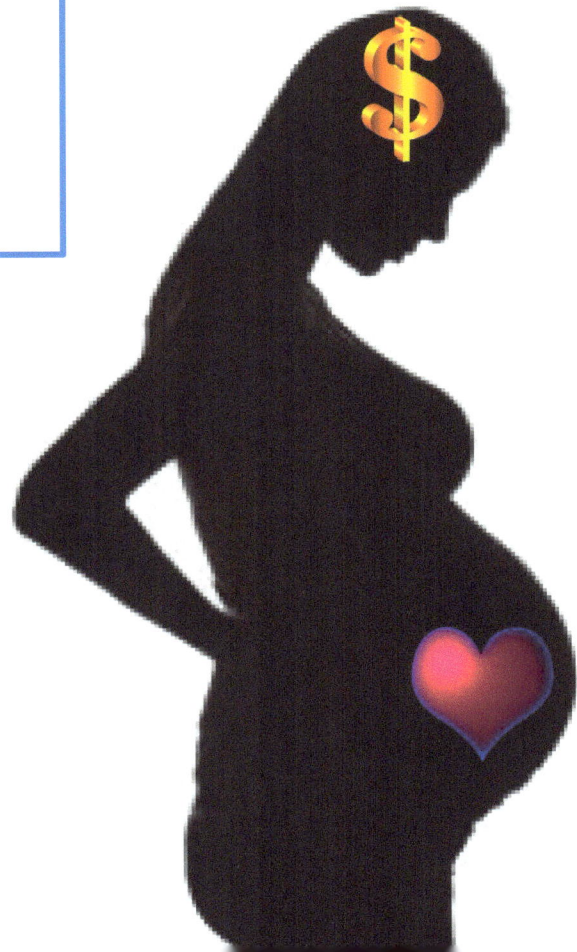

Combatting Relationship Concerns

✓ Be Ready for a
  Long-Term Healthy
  Relationship.

✓ Talk about
  everything.

✓ Engage in Good
  Conversation.

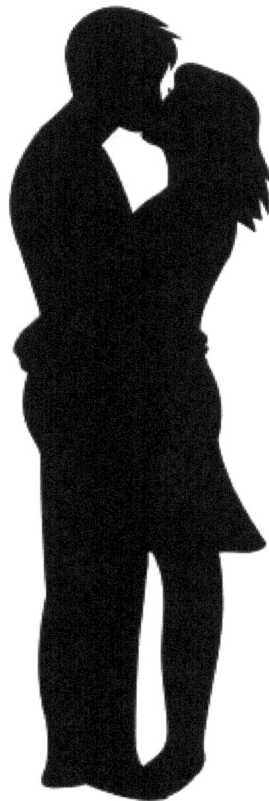

✓ Practice Good
  Communication
  Skills.

✓ Make Time for
  Each Other.

✓ Have Fun
  Together.

PREGNANCY
WiSHES

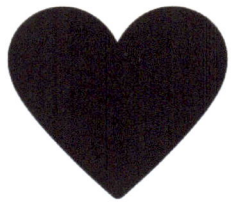

♥ Prenatal Affirmations ♥

- In the same way that new concerns can arise during the prenatal period, new wishes can arise as well!

- Affirmations are positive statements that are expressed in the present tense.

Examples:

"I welcome and love the changes in my body."

"My baby hears my laughter."

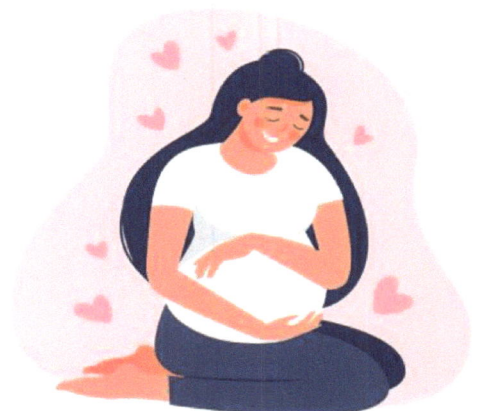

Prenatal Affirmations - Examples

I choose to **believe good things** about **pregnancy** **birth** and **motherhood**

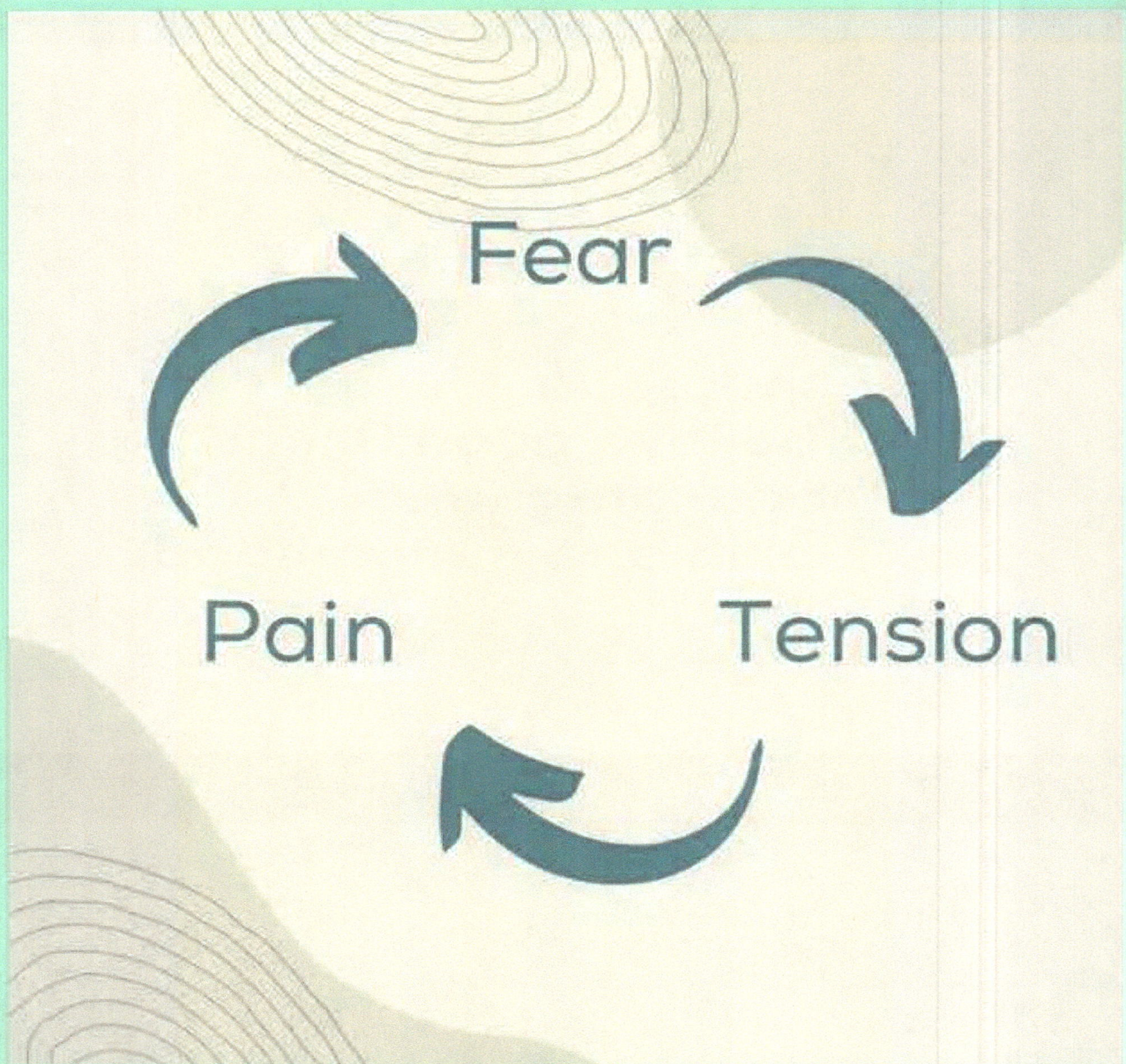

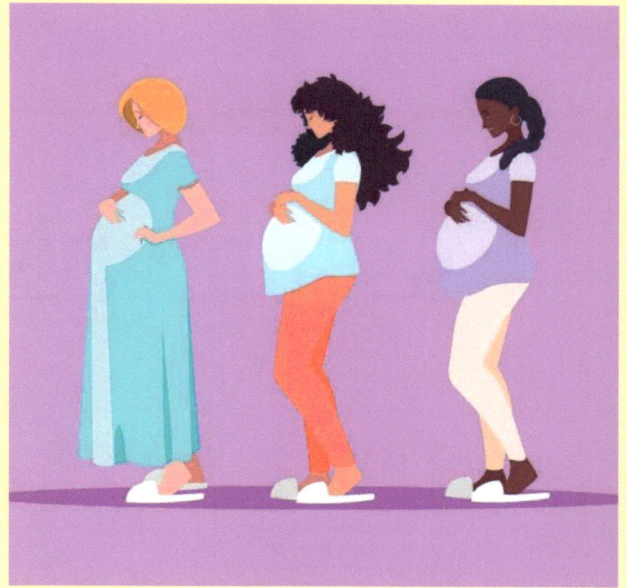

Breakout!

1. Enter your breakout group & re-introduce yourself.

2. Choose a Spokesperson.

3. Discuss one (or more) Prenatal Affirmation(s) that are meaningful

4. Have your Spokesperson share the group's thoughts with the class without disclosing who they were in a group with.

5. 5 minutes for activity.

Communicate and Connect

- **Talk to Your Baby Daily!**

- **Consider Ways You Can Communicate with your baby.**

- **Share Expectations, Hopes, Thoughts, Dreams and Feelings with Your Baby.**

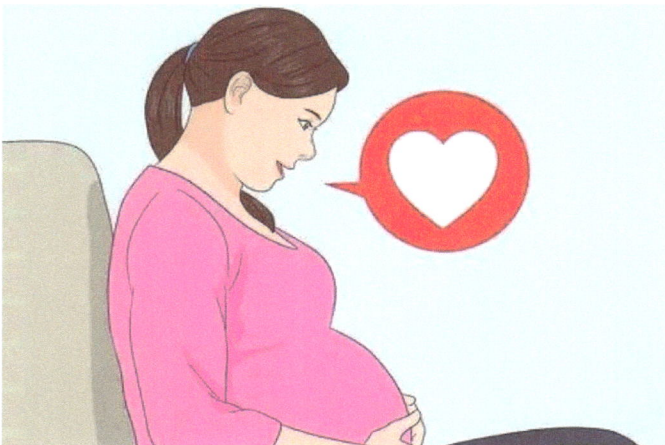

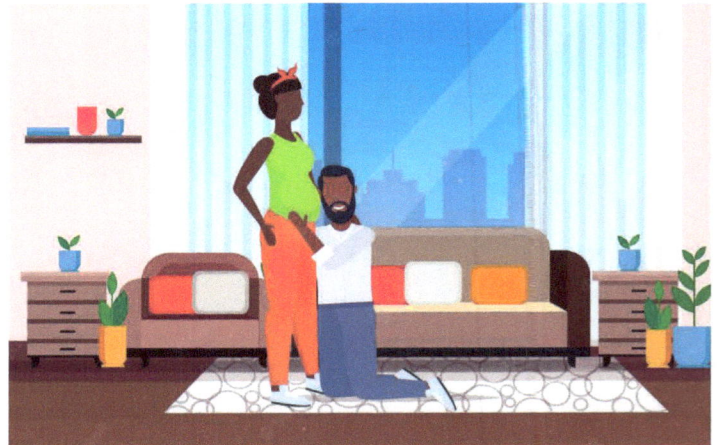

Connecting With Your Baby In The Womb

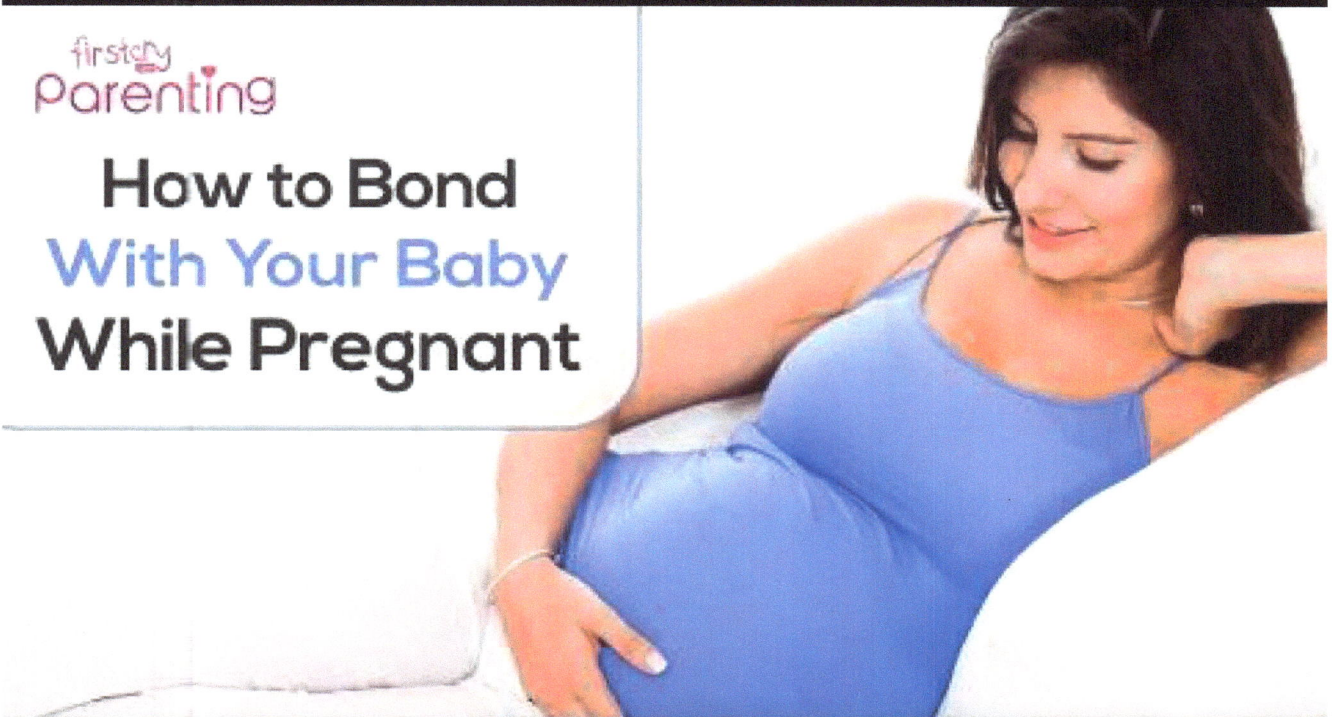

firsty Parenting

How to Bond With Your Baby While Pregnant

Connecting With Your Baby In The Womb: **Affirmations**

Connecting to my Baby
in the womb

**A Built To Birth
Guided Meditation**

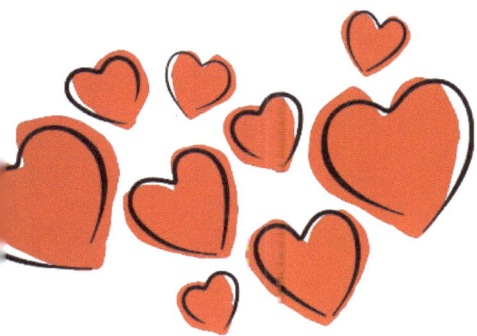

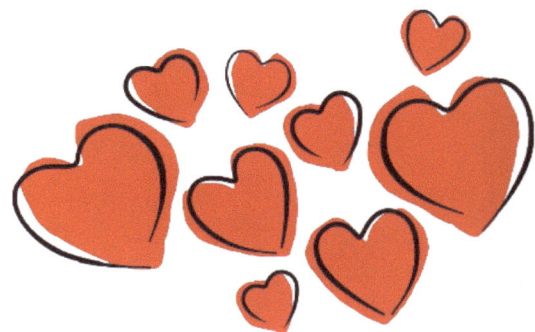

Each labor contraction is caused by a wave of **Oxytocin** (the love hormone) coursing through your body. So, very literally, each birthing surge is a surge of love. Allow yourself to meet each surge with the same warmth, intimacy and acceptance that you would experience during a kiss or a loving embrace.
~Lauralyn Curtis

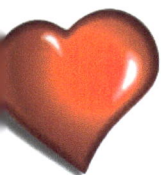

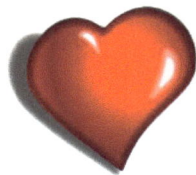

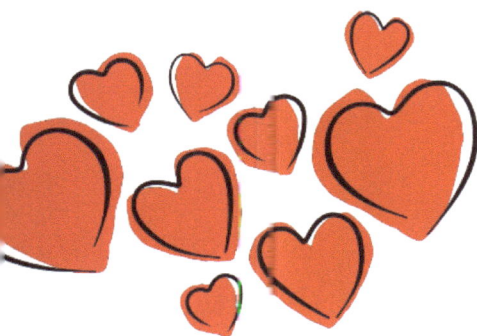

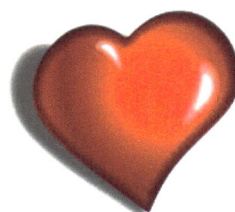

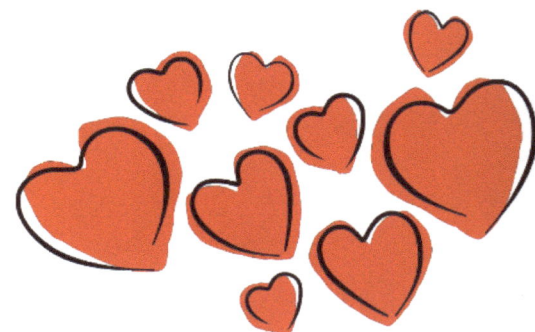

Connect with your Baby, Today.

Prenatal Nurturing & Nutrition

session2

Madonna Igah-Okoro, Ph.D, M.P.H., B.S.

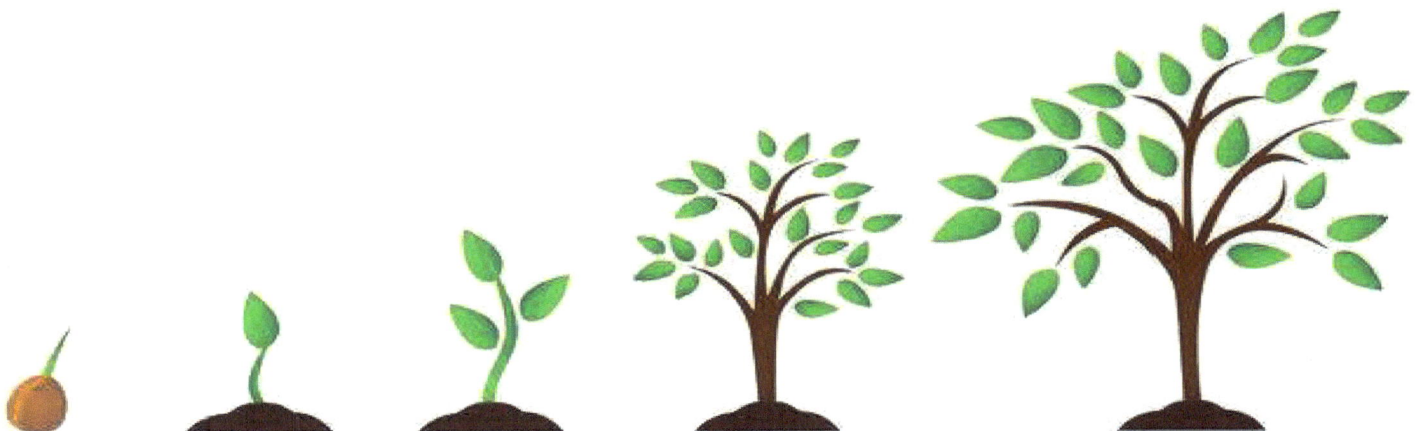

Today's Lesson Topics:

- Changes during pregnancy.

- Womb Anatomy.

- Pregnancy Trimesters.

- Baby's Development.

- Mom's Development.

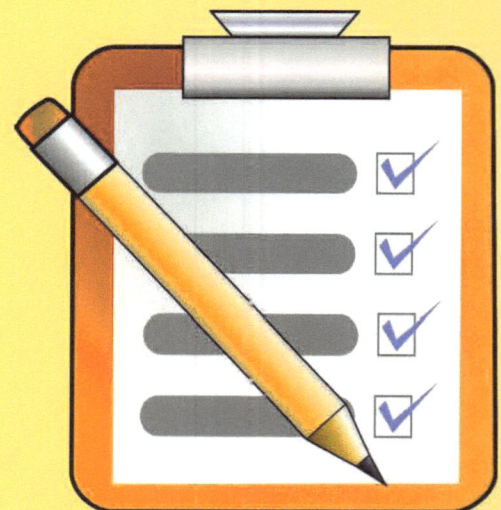

Just as a woman's heart knows how and when to pump, her lungs to inhale, and her hand to pull back from fire, so she knows when and how to give birth.

~ Virginia Di Orio

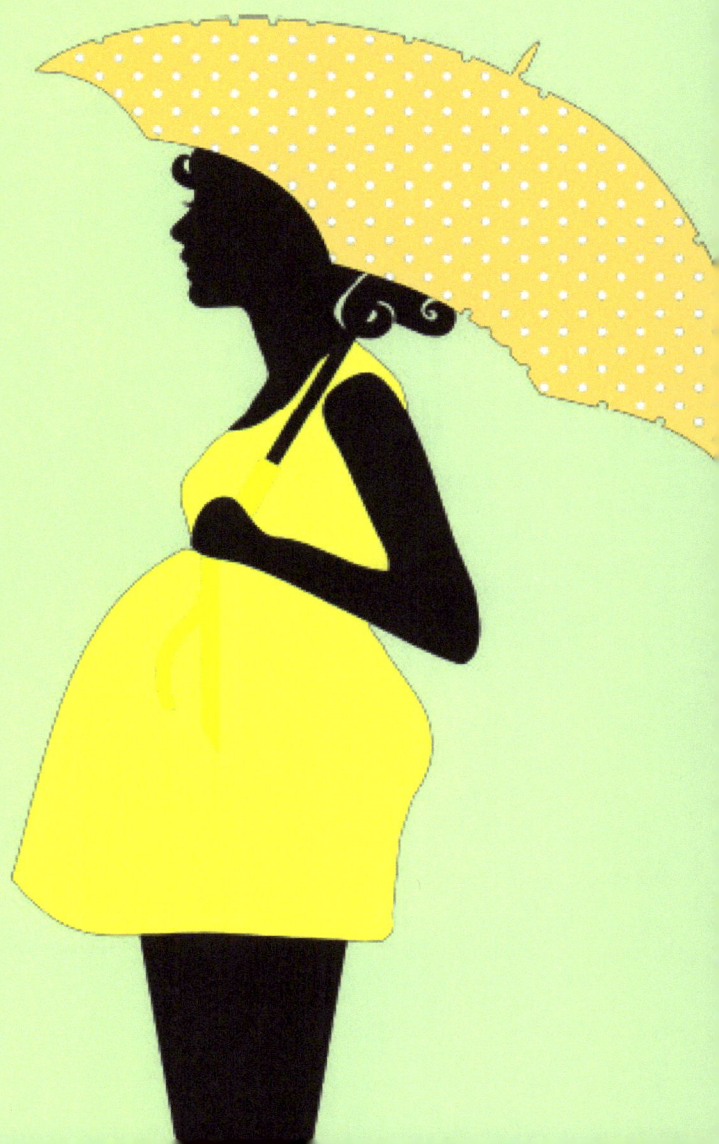

Changes During Pregnancy

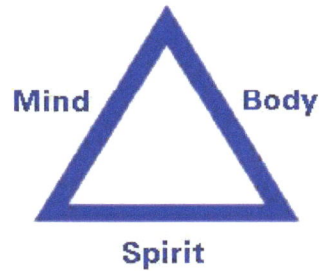

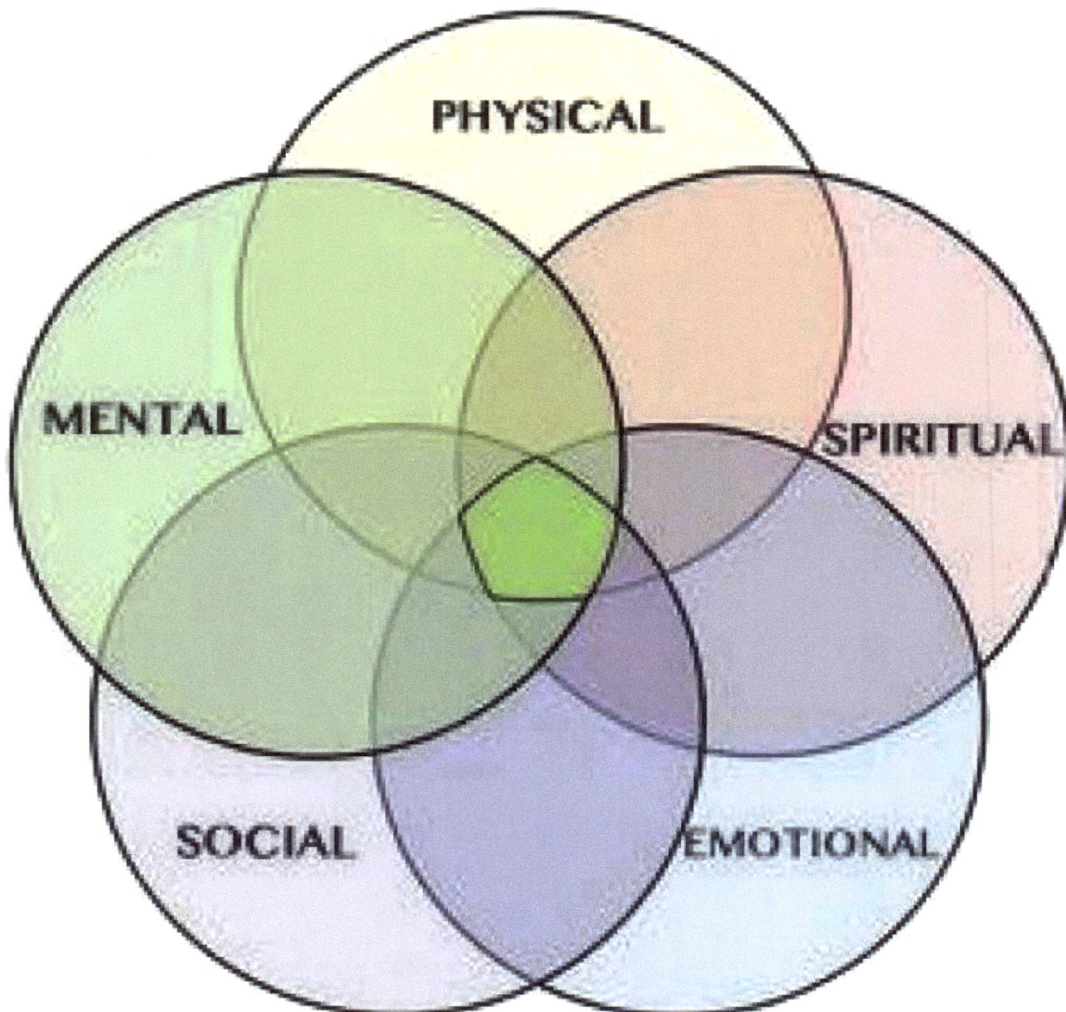

Mind
Body
Spirit

PHYSICAL

MENTAL

SPIRITUAL

SOCIAL

EMOTIONAL

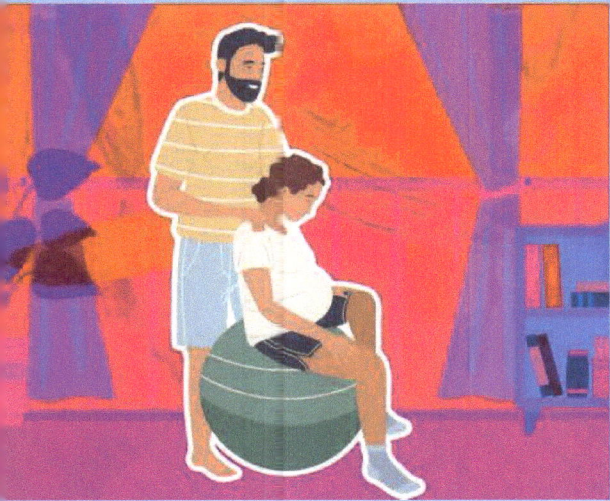

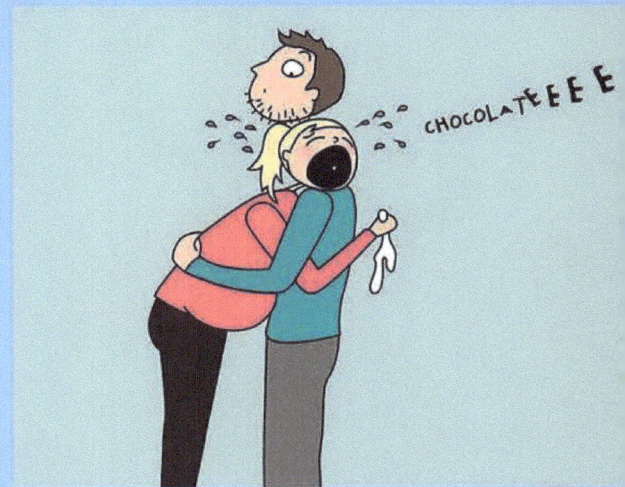

S
U
P
P
O
R
T

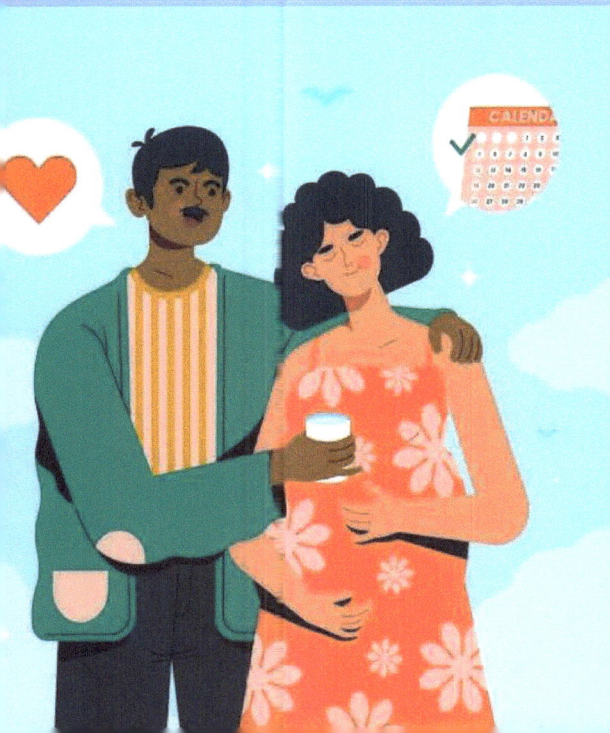

CHOCOLATEEEE

Never Alone ♡

All I need is within me.
I am stronger than I seem.
I am braver than I think.
I have unshakable faith.
Miracles are taking place.
I am done complaining.
I am grateful.
I appreciate my life.

You are Strong

Stay Calm and Focus

Breathe and Relax

You're the Best

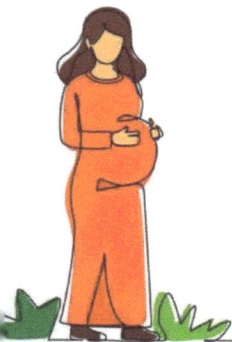

Have You Noticed?

- **Changes in Sexual Activity?**

- **Changes in Communication between you and your partner?**

- **Changes in perceptions of self, and others?**

- **Changes in priorities?**

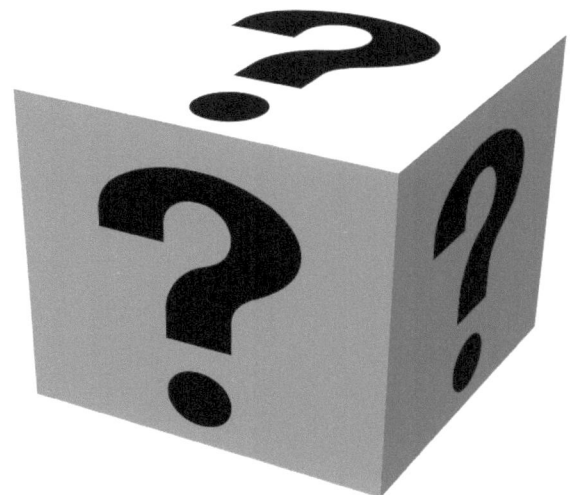

Breakout!

1. Enter your breakout
   group & re-introduce
   yourself. (name and pregnancy trimester)

2. Choose a Spokesperson.

3. To your comfort level: Discuss what changes you have already noticed (from you and/or your partner).

4. Would you say that the changes were physical, emotional, mental, spiritual, or social?

5. Have your Spokesperson share the
   group's thoughts with the class **without disclosing who they were in a group with.**

6. 5 minutes for activity.

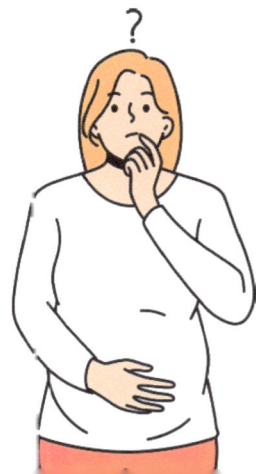

Common Physical Changes

- Breasts Enlarge
- Morning Sickness
- Fatigue
- New Energy Levels
- Body Temperature

- Indigestion
- Heartburn
- Breathlessness

- Vision Changes
- Constipation
- Urinary Problems
- Stretch Marks
- Swelling

- Acne
- Weight Gain

Emotional Changes

- **Hormonal Changes:**

  — **Prolactin**
  — **Progesterone**
  — **Estrogen**
  — **Relaxin**
  — **Oxytocin**

- **Symptoms:**

  -Moodiness
  -Memory Loss
  -Vivid Dreams
  -Identity Crisis
  -Stress

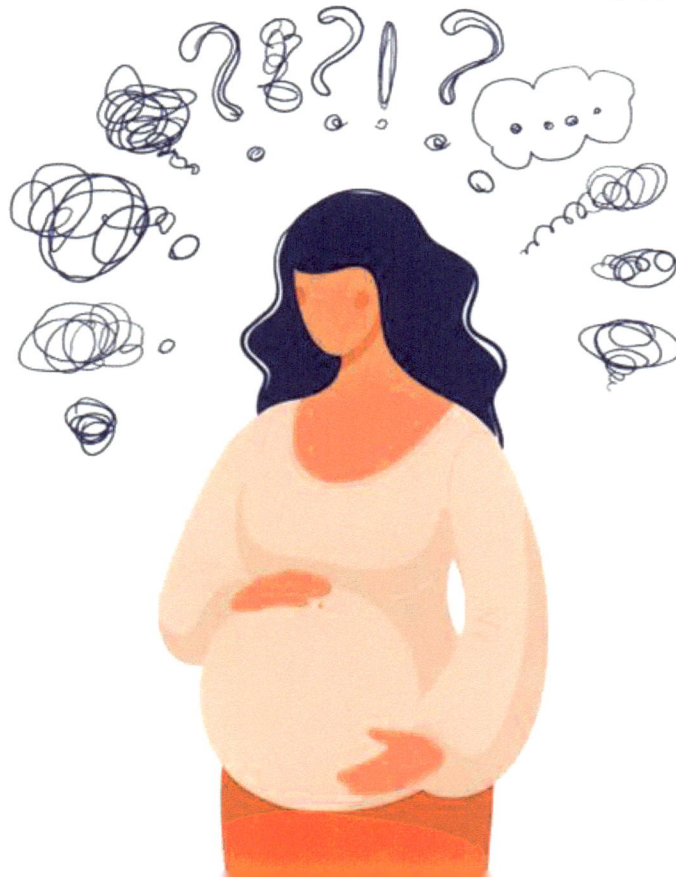

Social Changes

❑ Significant Relationships

❑ Friends and Family

❑ Acquaintances and Strangers

❑ Common Interest Groups

❑ Sexual Relationships

Physical Approaches

- Listen to your body.

- Stretch away tension.

- Learn relaxation skills.
  - Breathing Exercises
  - Meditation
  - Muscle relaxation for stress relief
  - Visualization meditation for stress relief (video)

- Get adequate sleep.

Directed Visualization

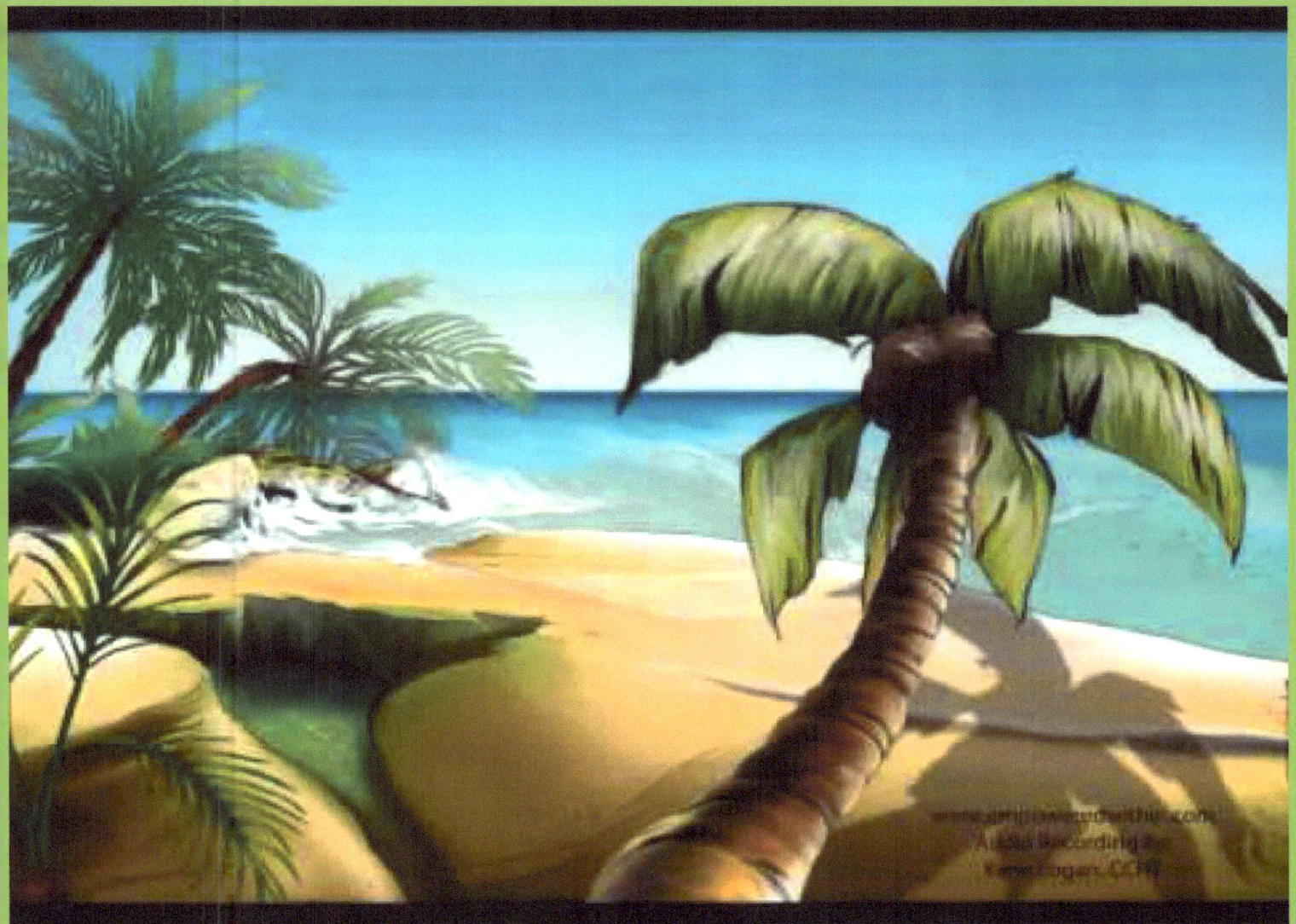

Mental Approaches

- Adopt a new attitude.

- Increase self-worth.

- Set realistic expectations.

- Keep a positive outlook.

- Improve your communication skills.

- Leave work at work.

- Get organized.

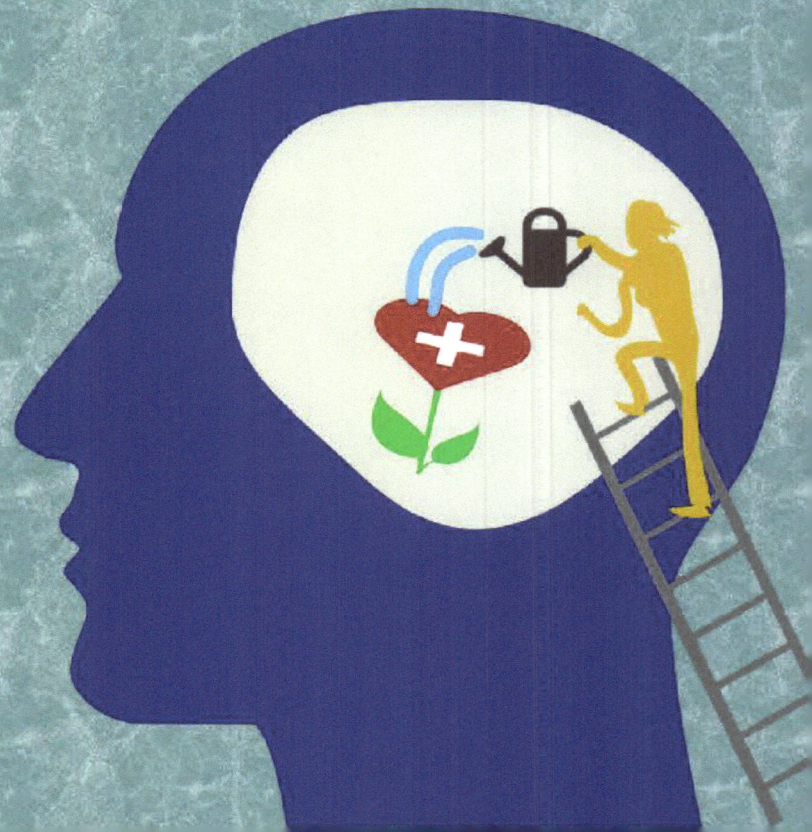

Social Approaches

- Develop a support network.

- Develop a social life.

- Volunteer your time.

- Develop a sense of humor.

- Develop hobbies.

Pregnancy and Sleep

- Sleep problems are common during pregnancy.

- Pregnant women are more likely to suffer from sleep disturbances.

  - Some common sleep-related disorders during pregnancy include:
    - insomnia
    - restless legs syndrome
    - obstructive sleep apnea
    - night-time gastroesophageal reflux disease

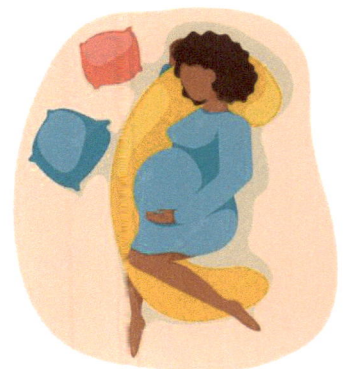

Sleep is Very Important, Especially Now!

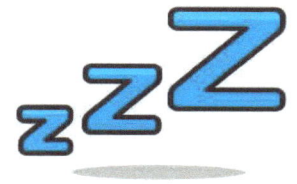

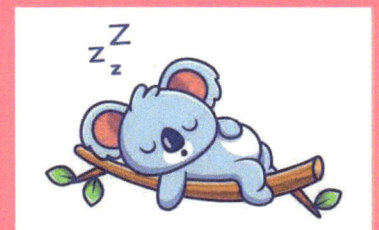

"Pregnancy is the only time when you can do nothing at all and still be productive."

— EVAN ESAR

Pregnancy Sleep-Positions

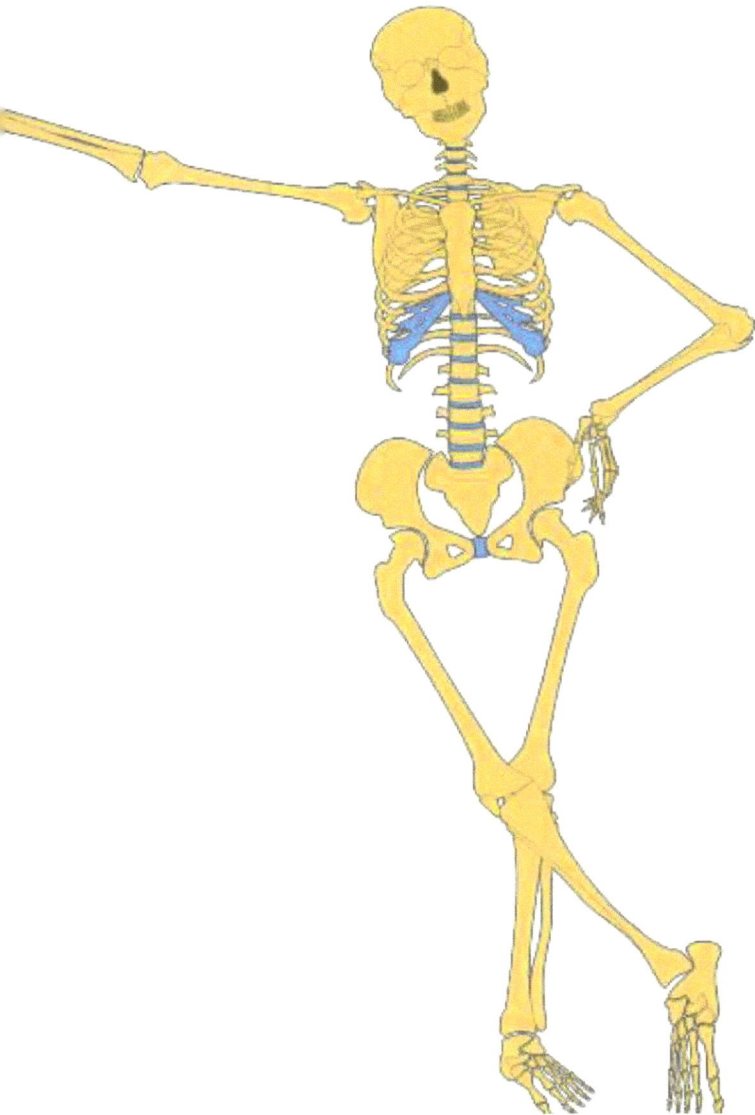

Taking a Closer Look at the Womb

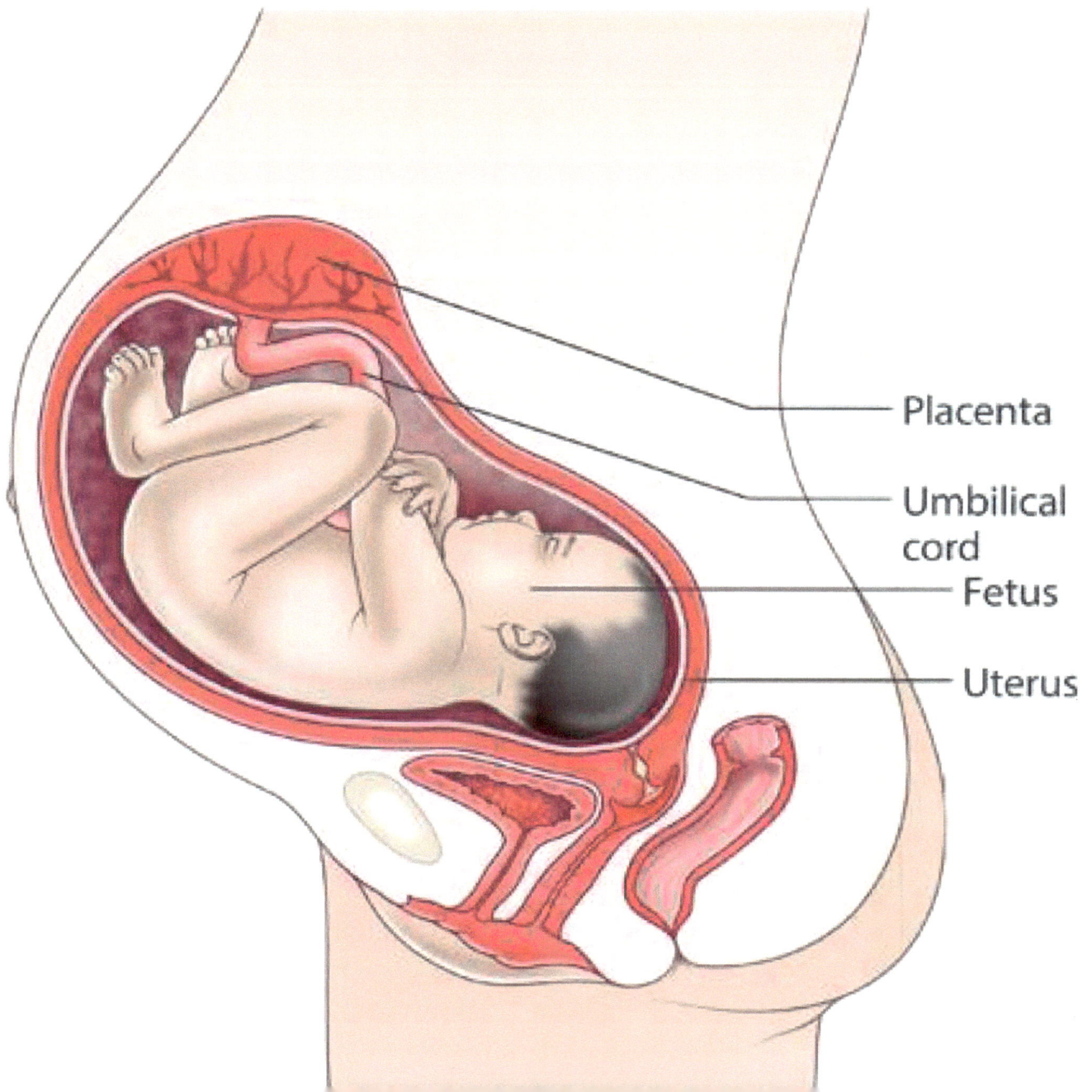

Placenta

Umbilical cord

Fetus

Uterus

EMBRYONIC DEVELOPMENT

I TRIMESTER

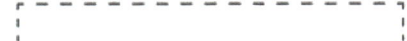

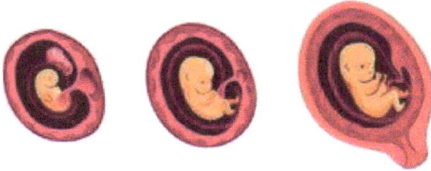

1 MONTH   2 MONTH   3 MONTH

II TRIMESTER

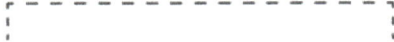

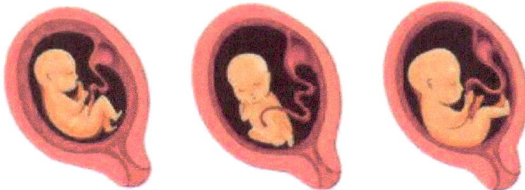

4 MONTH   5 MONTH   6 MONTH

III TRIMESTER

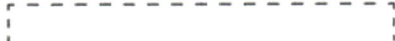

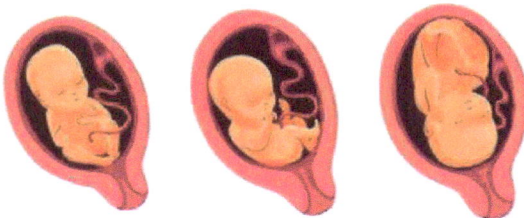

7 MONTH   8 MONTH   9 MONTH

Baby's Development in Womb

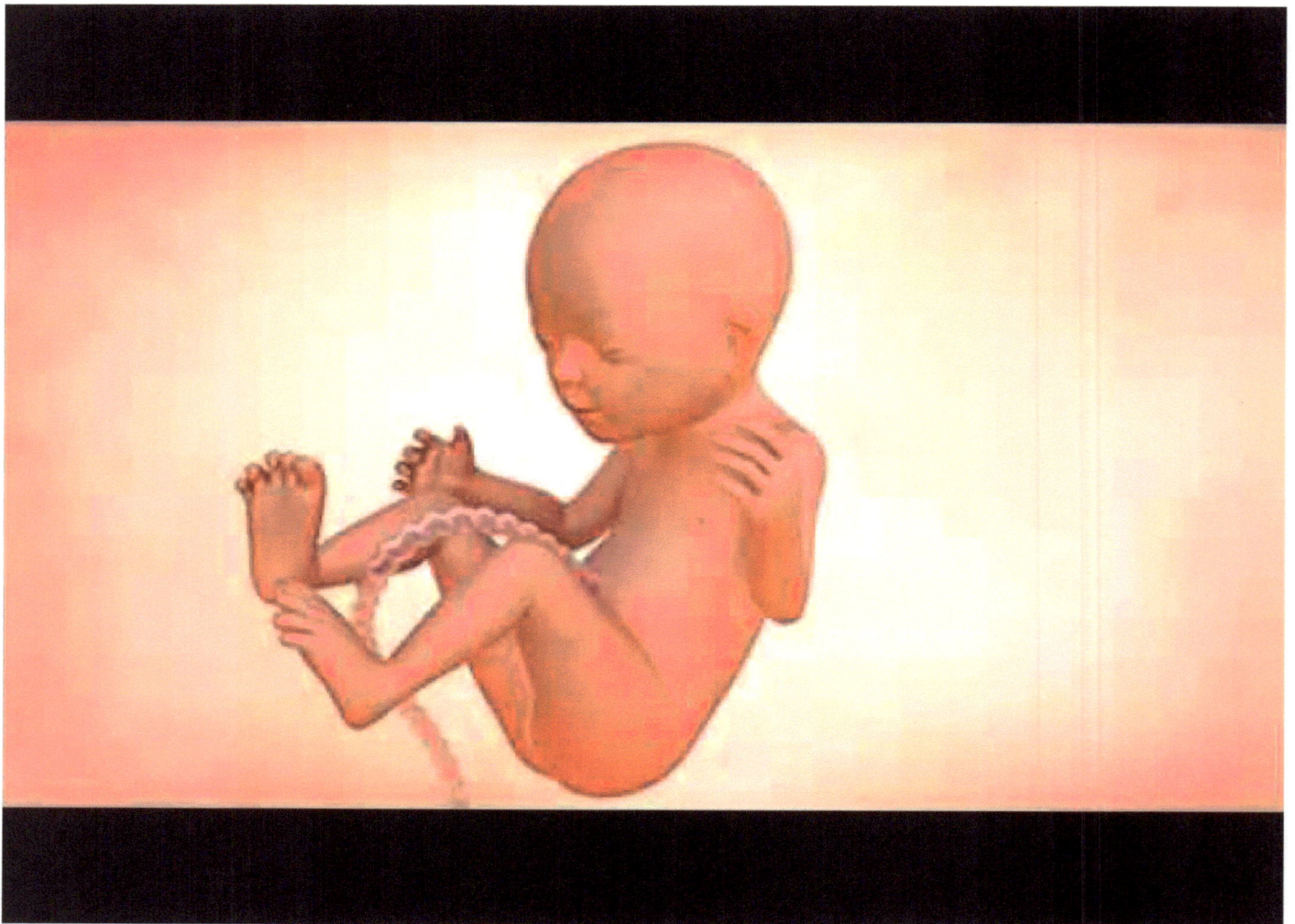

Mom's Prenatal Development:

PREGNANCY
STAGES

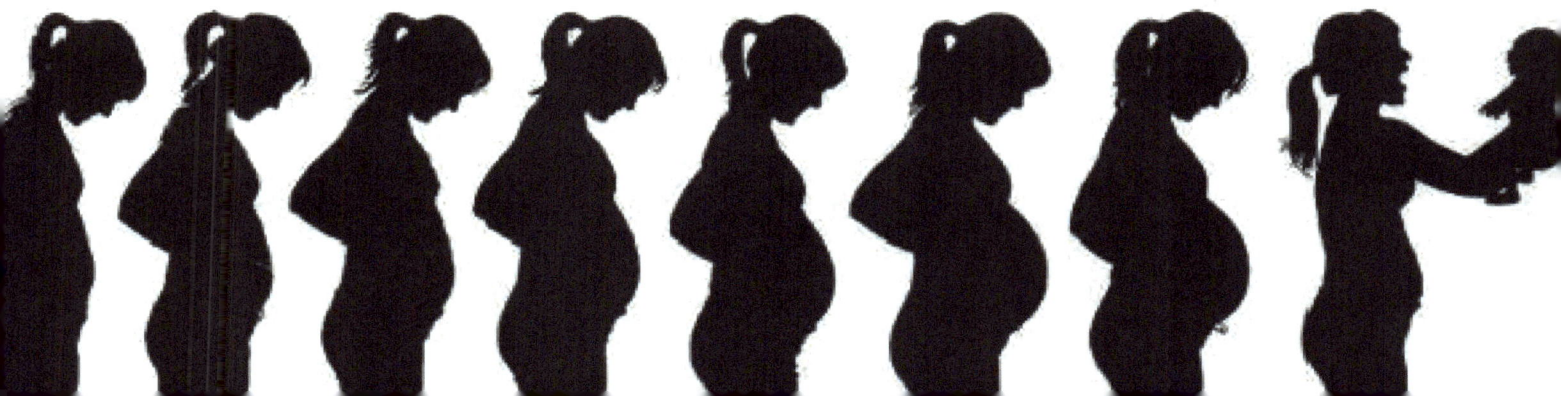

What to Expect in Your 1st Trimester

First

- nausea and vomiting
- cravings and aversions
- heightened sense of smell
- mood swings

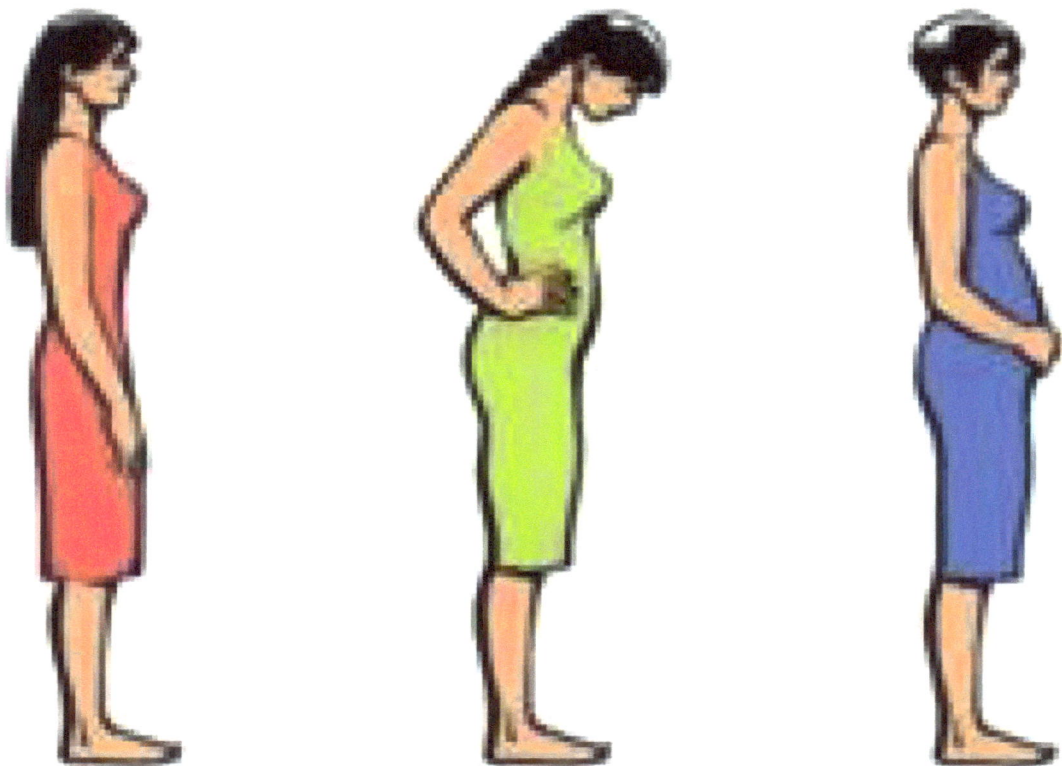

What to Expect in Your 2nd Trimester

Second

- round ligament pains
- nipple changes
- stretch marks
- feeling the baby moving

What to Expect in Your 3rd Trimester

Third

- strong kicks from the baby
- swollen feet
- leaking from the breasts
- frequent urination

Mom's Pregnancy Development

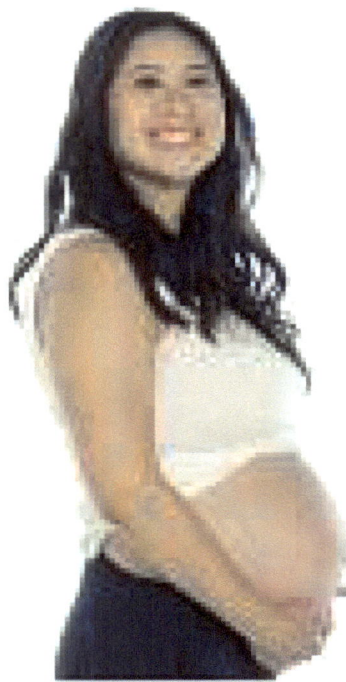
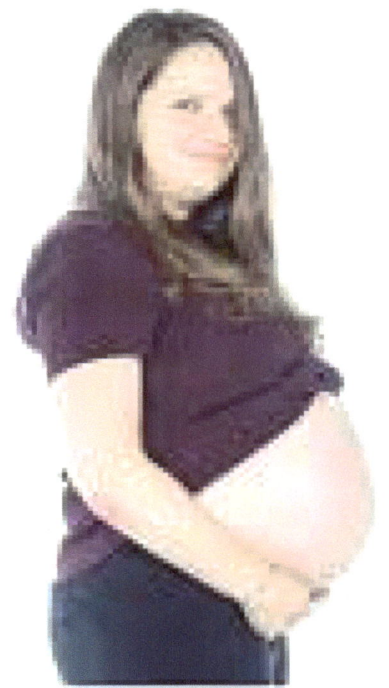

16 WEEKS   33 WEEKS   40 WEEKS

Mom's Pregnancy Development

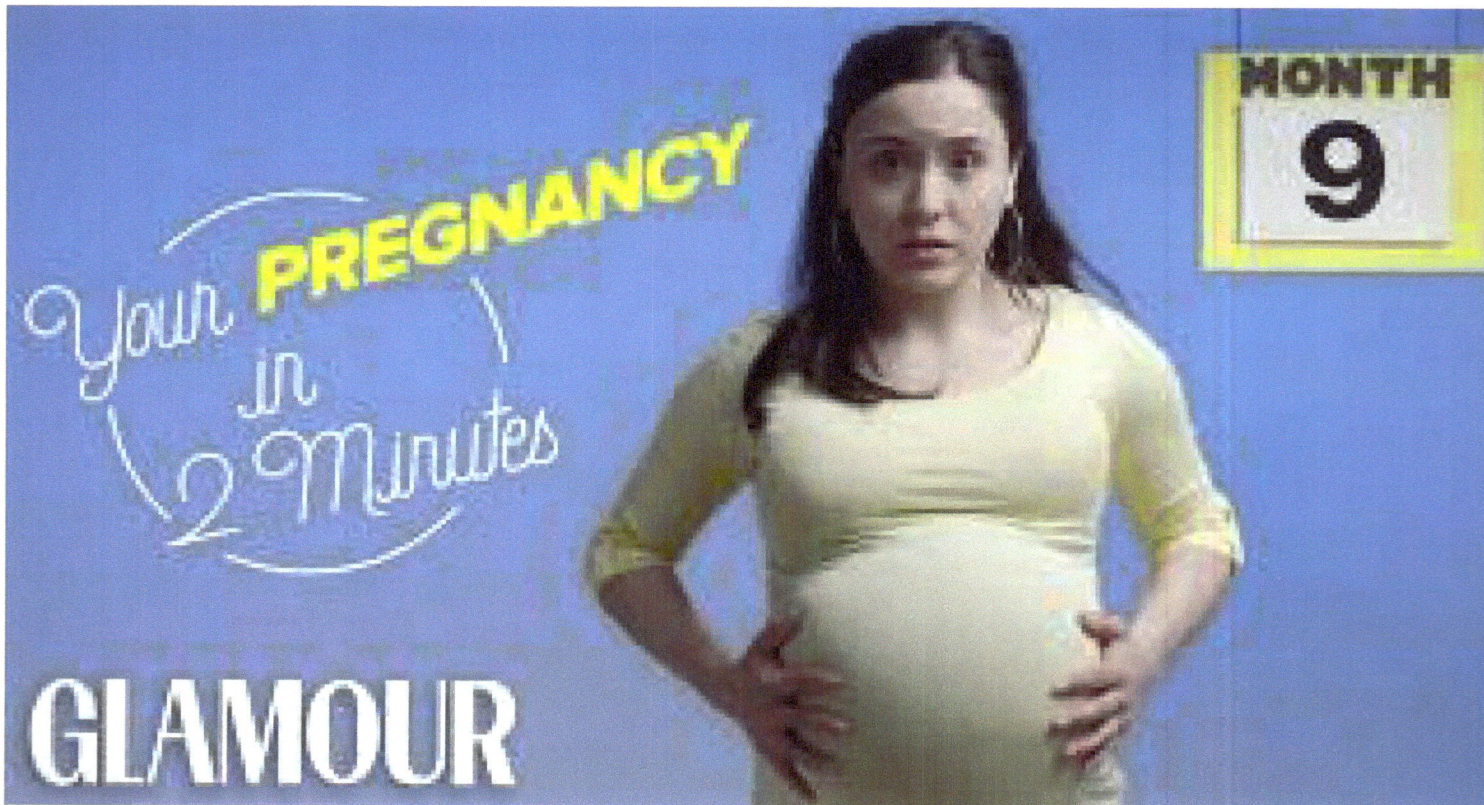

Pregnancy Development

Your Body is Working Very Hard to Serve You and Your Baby!

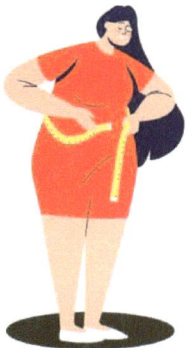

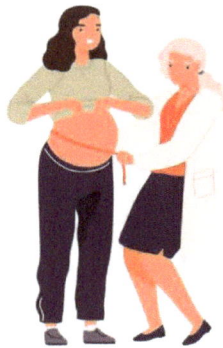

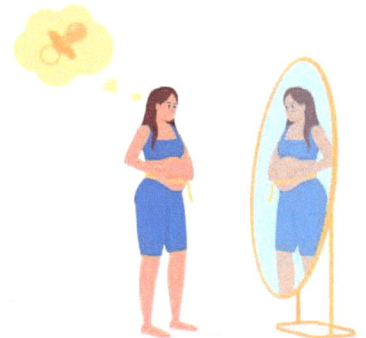

What Happens to Your Organs?

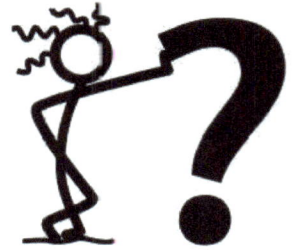

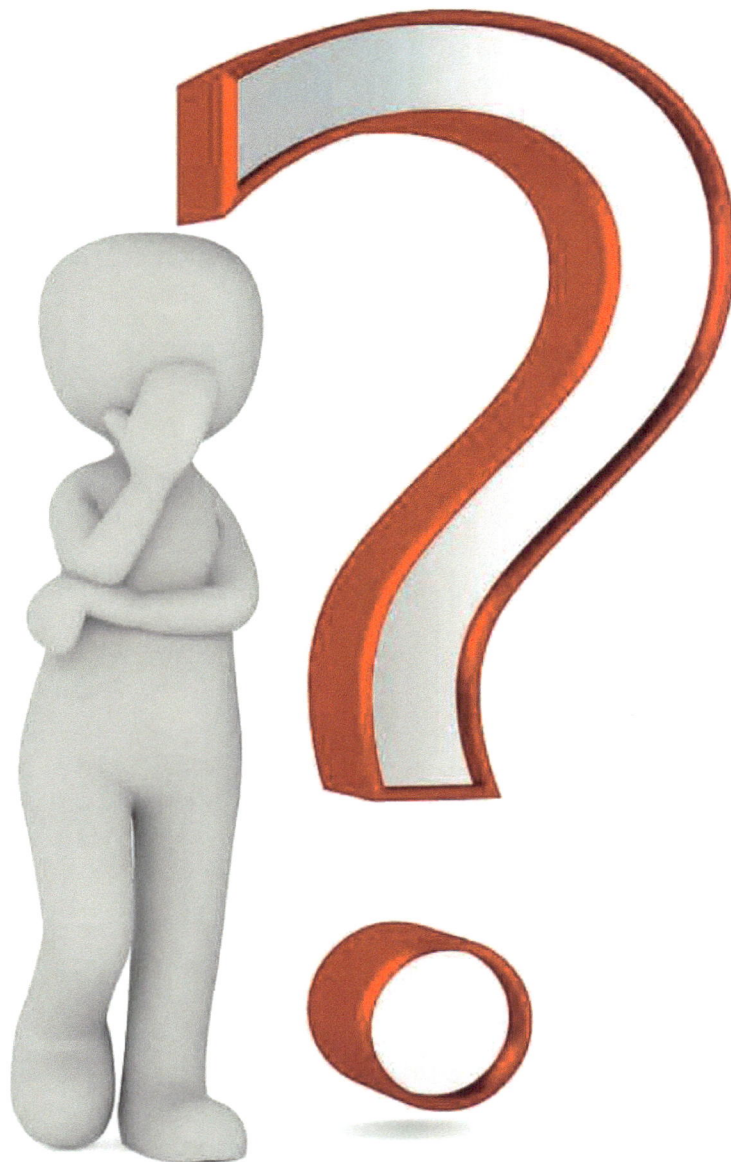

Pregnancy Development

- **What happens to your organs during pregnancy?**

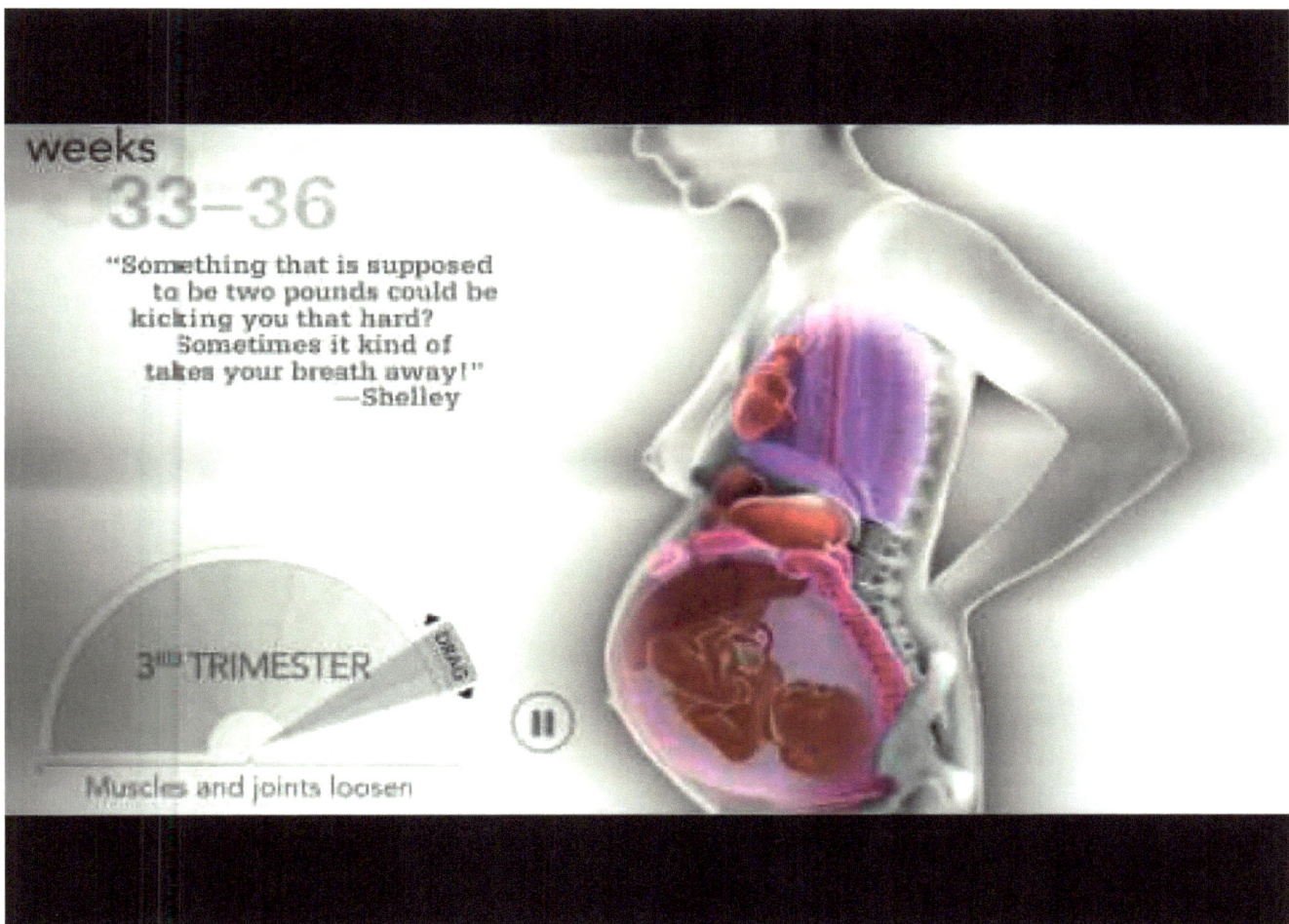

weeks
33–36

"Something that is supposed
to be two pounds could be
kicking you that hard?
Sometimes it kind of
takes your breath away!"
—Shelley

3RD TRIMESTER

Muscles and joints loosen

MY
AMAZING
BODY

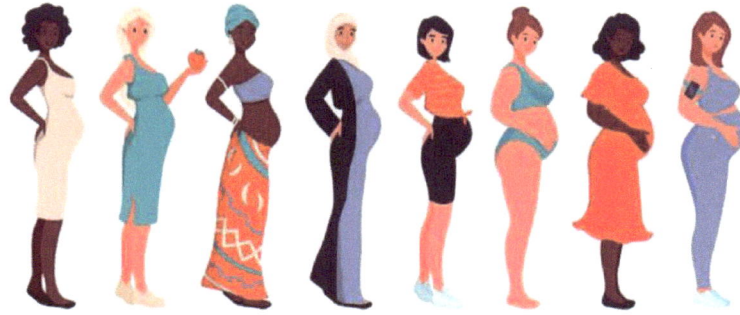

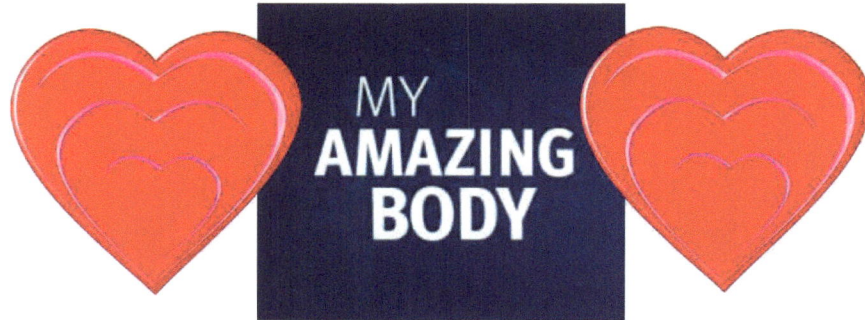

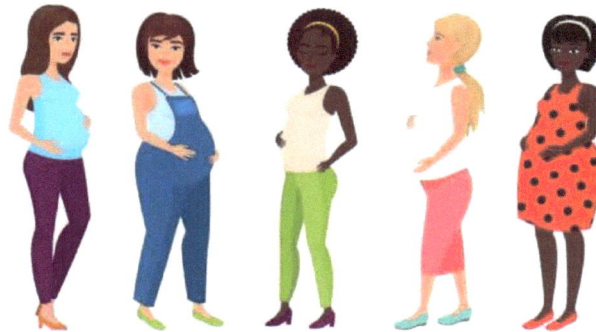

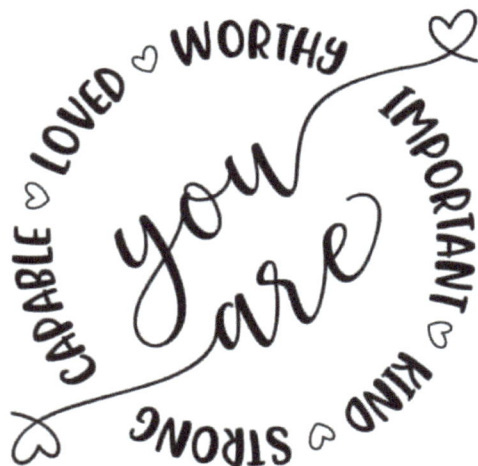

YOU
are capable of
amazing
things.

CAPABLE ♡ LOVED ♡ WORTHY
you IMPORTANT
are
STRONG ♡ KIND

Show Appreciation for your Baby and your Body, Today.

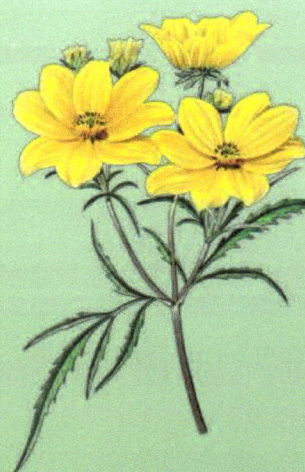

Prenatal Nurturing & Nutrition

session3

Madonna Igah-Okoro, Ph.D, M.P.H., B.S.

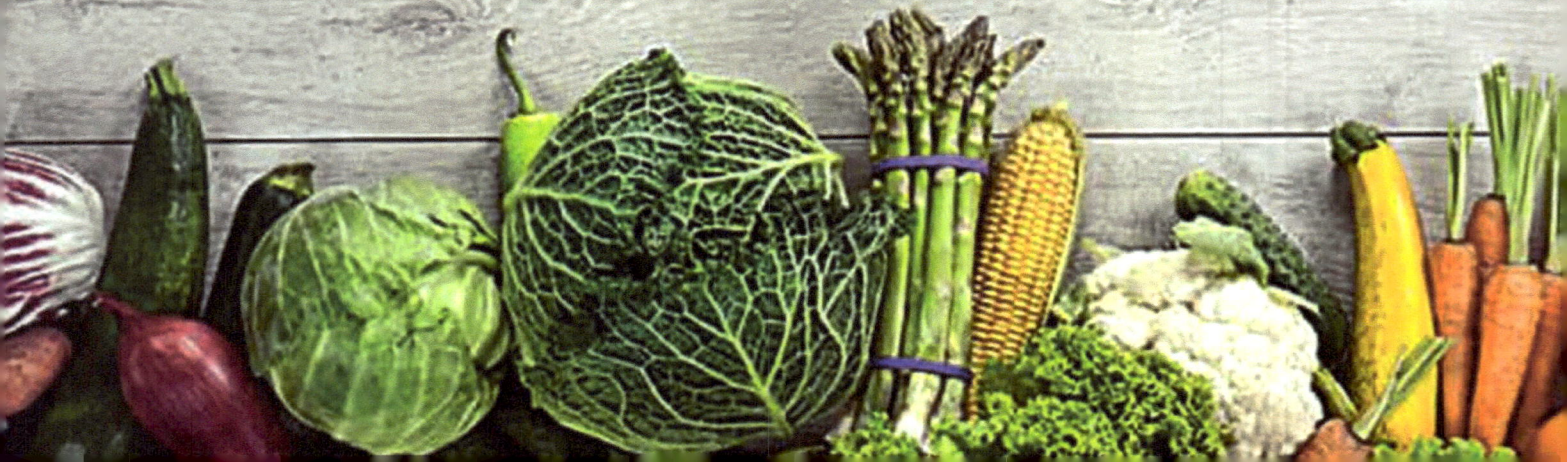

Today's Lesson Topics:

- Dietary needs during pregnancy.

- Challenges with achieving proper nutrition.

- Stress, and foods that help.

- Smoking and Alcohol Usage during pregnancy.

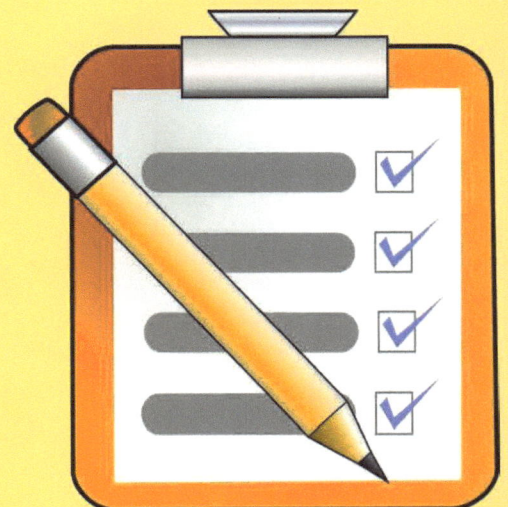

One of the first and most essential ways a woman begins to exercise her role as a mother to her baby is by paying attention to what she eats while she is pregnant.

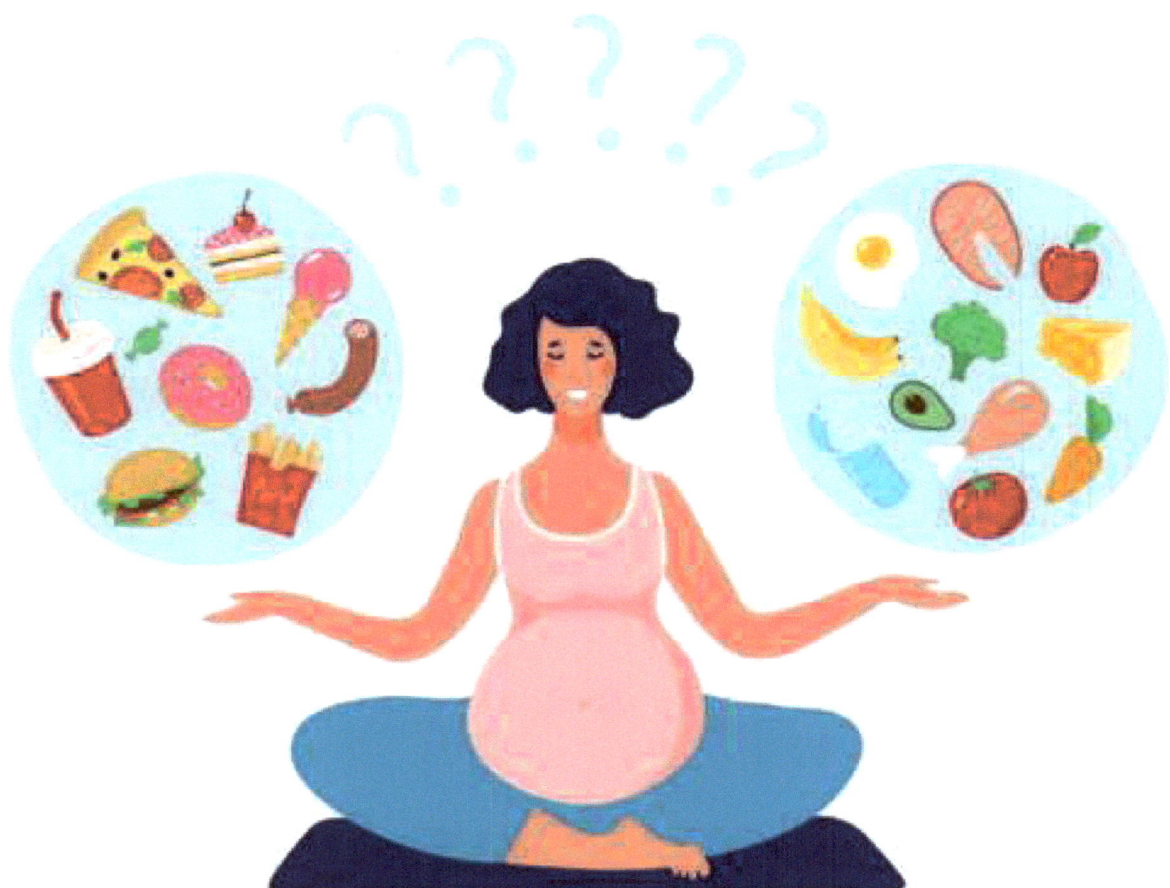

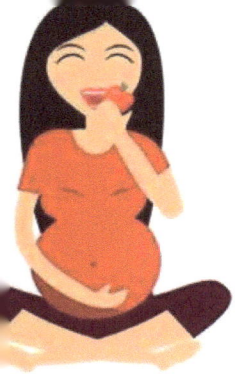

Improve Your Diet!

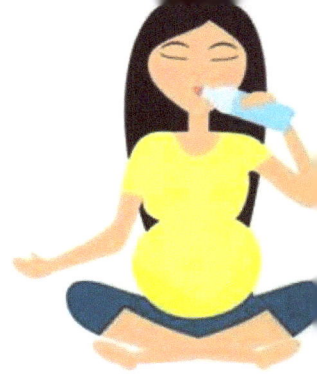

- Your Diet is very important, especially right now!

    -Sometimes we know what we should eat, however we don't take seriously the practice of eating healthy meals.

    -Balance is the key.

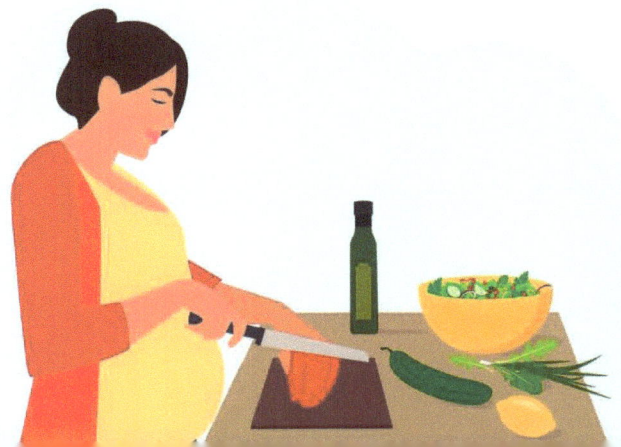

Basic Prenatal Nutrition: My Pregnancy Plate

My Pregnancy Plate

Choose large portions of a variety of non-starchy vegetables, such as leafy greens, broccoli, carrots, peppers or cabbage.

Choose small amounts of healthy oils (olive and canola) for cooking or to flavor foods. Nuts, seeds and avocados contain healthy fats.

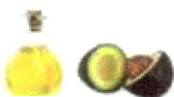

Choose a variety of whole fruits. Limit juice and dried fruits.

Fruit is great for snacks and dessert, too.

Aim for at least 30 minutes of walking or another physical activity each day.

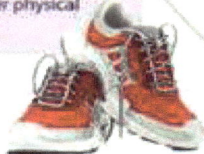

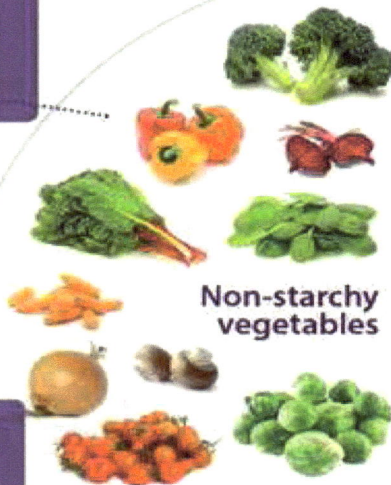

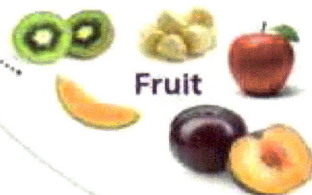

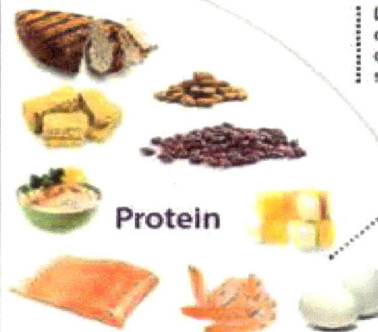

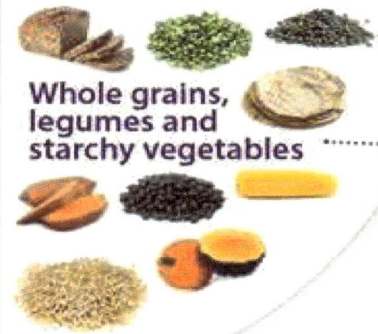

Choose 2 to 3 servings of nonfat or 1% milk or yogurt (cow, soy or almond). A serving is 8 oz. Choose yogurt with less than 15 g of sugar per serving.

Drink mainly water, decaf tea or decaf coffee and avoid sugary beverages.

Choose protein sources such as poultry, beans, nuts, low-mercury seafood, eggs, tofu or low-fat cheese. Limit red meat and avoid cold cuts and other processed meats.

Choose whole grains, such as whole wheat bread or pasta, brown rice, quinoa or oats and other healthy starches like beans, lentils, sweet potatoes or acorn squash. Limit white bread, white rice and fried potatoes.

Non-starchy vegetables

Protein

Fruit

Whole grains, legumes and starchy vegetables

OREGON HEALTH & SCIENCE UNIVERSITY

Risky Foods

Stay away from:

- Undercooked foods
- Unpasteurized drinks
- Soft cheeses
- Lunch meats and hot dogs
-
- Fatty/Salty/Sugary Foods

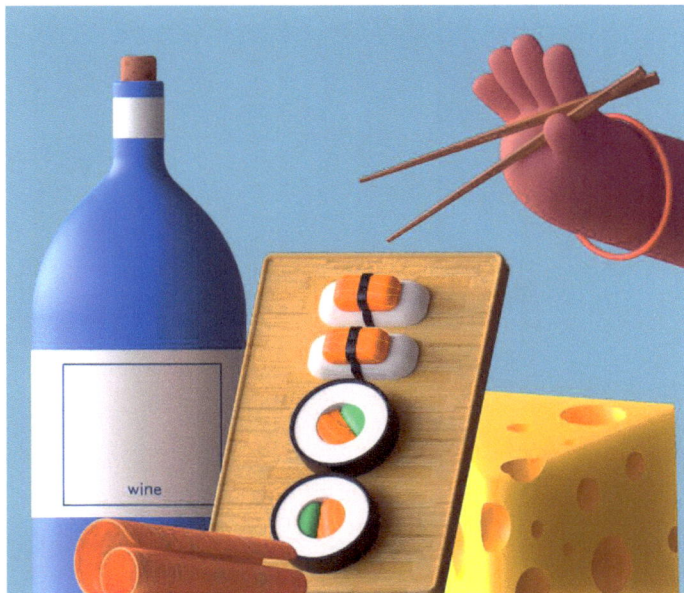

! Extra Nutrients Are Needed !

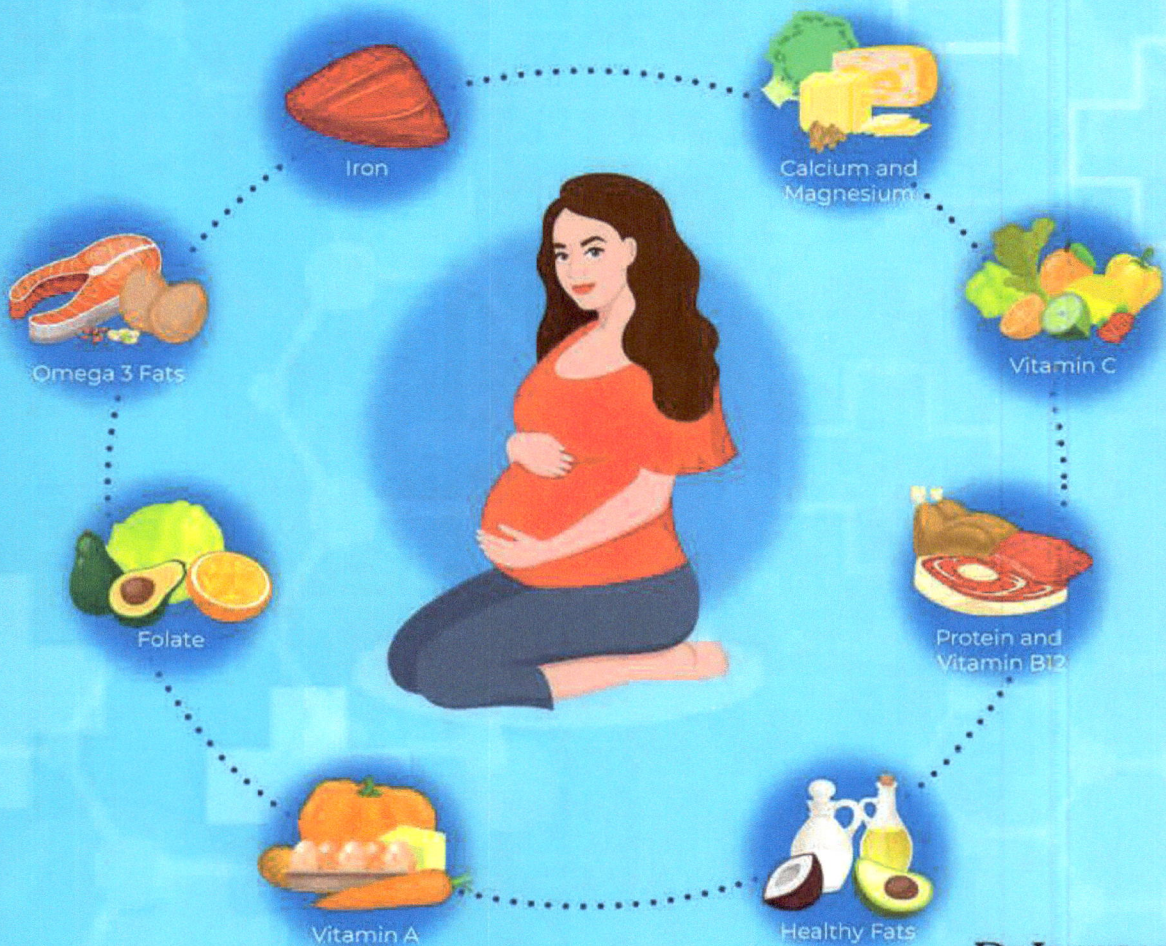

Your Baby's Prenatal Health:

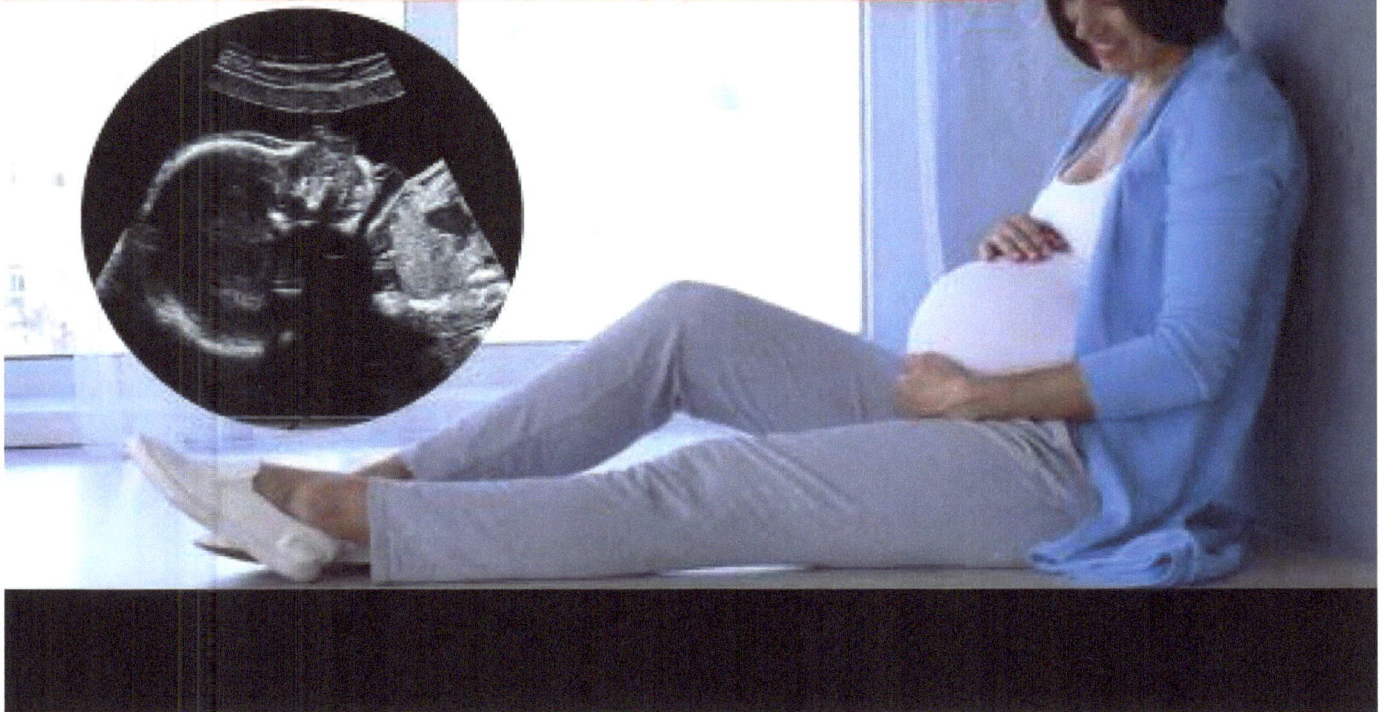

Breakout!

1. Enter your breakout group & re-introduce yourself.

2. Choose a Spokesperson.

3. Discuss whether you have been experiencing any pregnancy food cravings? If so, what are they?

4. Discuss which food(s)/food group(s) you would like to incorporate more in your pregnancy diet.

5. Have your Spokesperson share the group's thoughts with the class without disclosing who they were in a group with.

6. 5 minutes for activity.

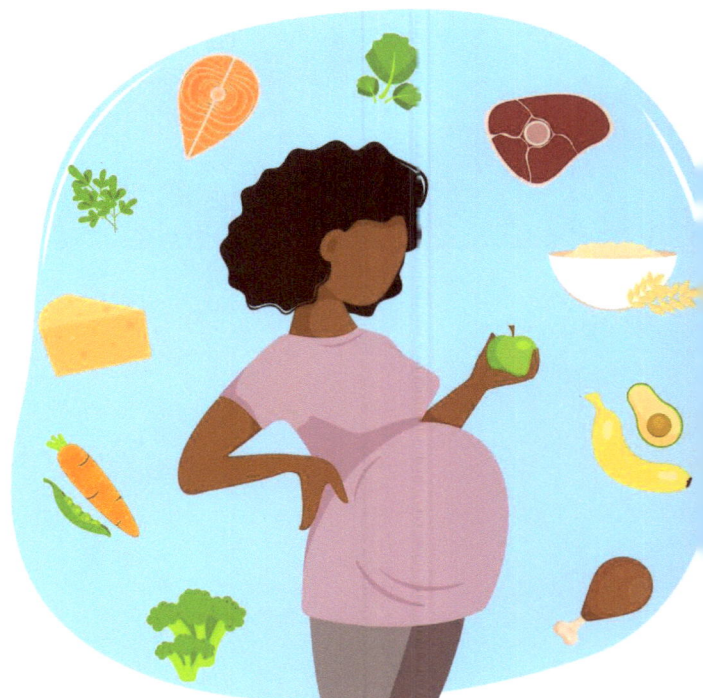

Factors that can Contribute to Poor Nutrition

- Poverty

- Work/Job

- Morning sickness

- Smoking/alcohol

- Living Status

- Dieting

- Food quality

- Weight/weight gain

- Previous pregnancy

- Stress

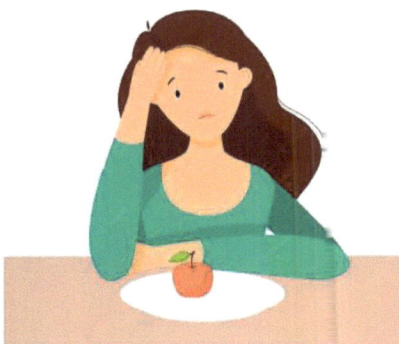

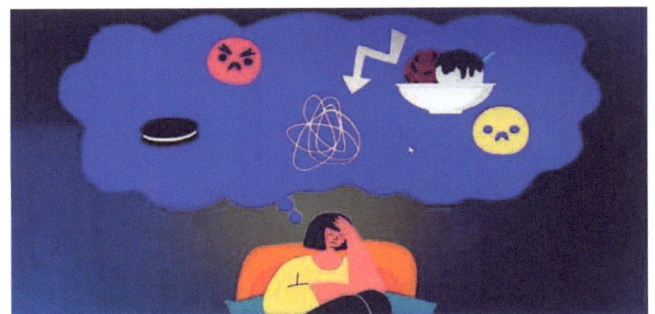

Stress During Pregnancy

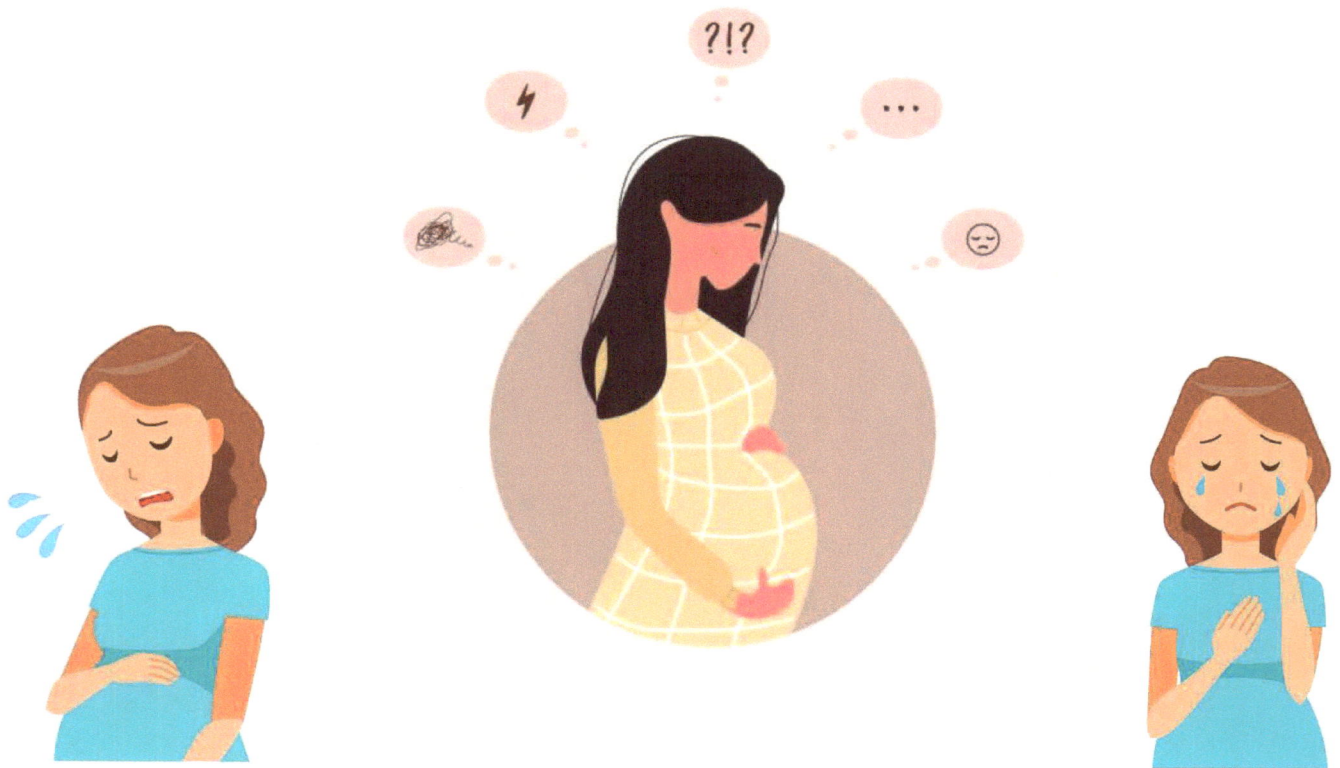

Stress-Busting Foods

- Stress-busting foods can help with stress management.

- Comfort foods can have a immediate calming effect.

- A healthy diet can help counter the impact(s) of stress.

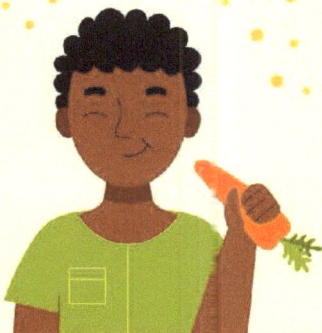 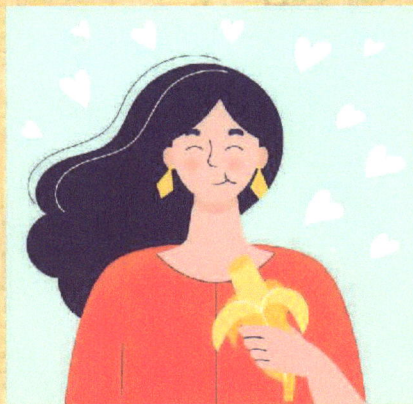 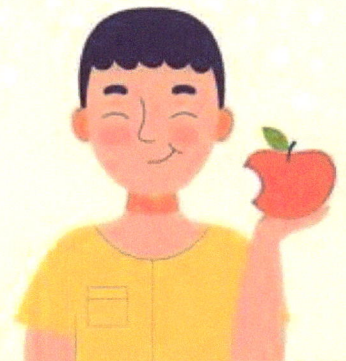

Complex Carbs

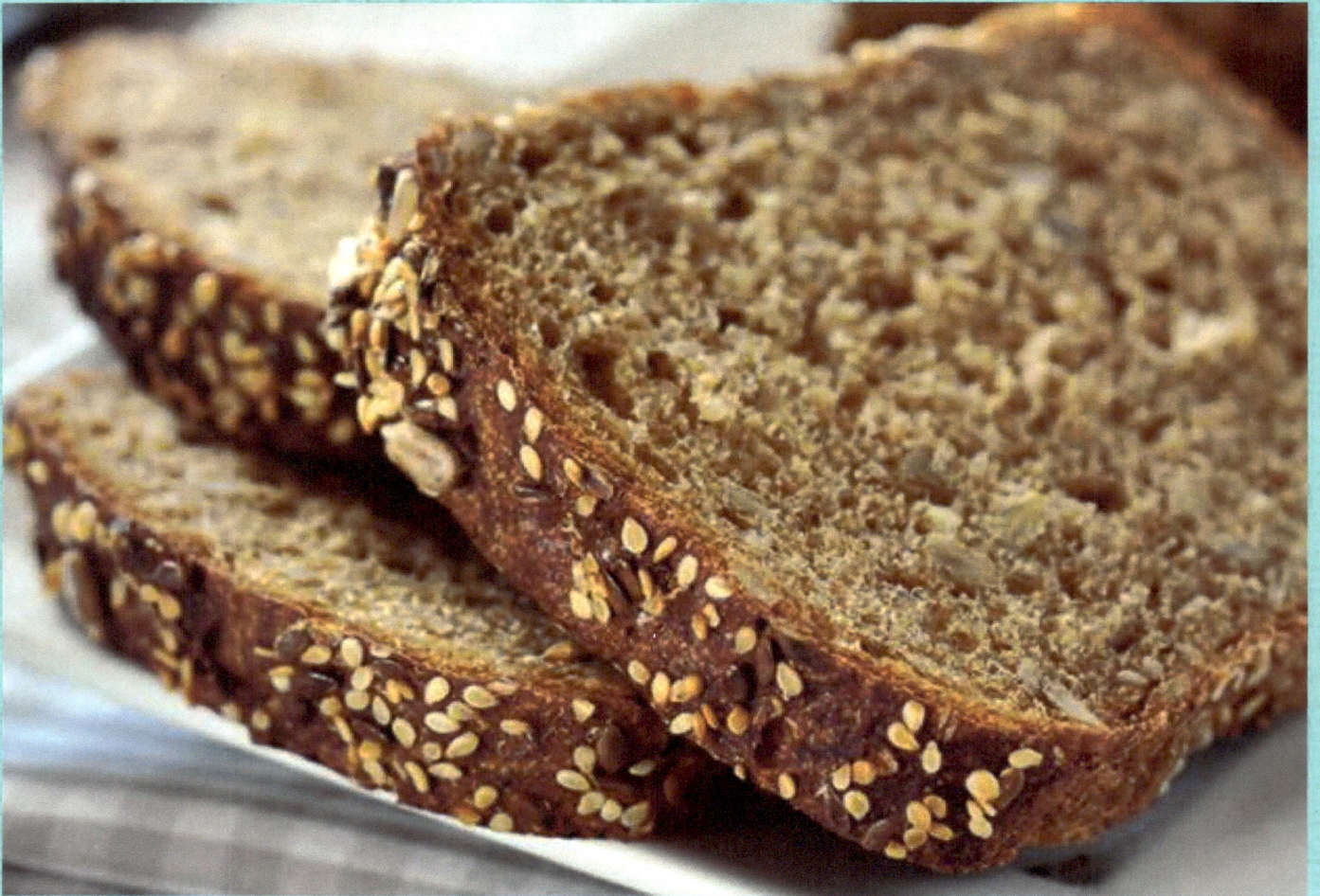

Simple Carbs

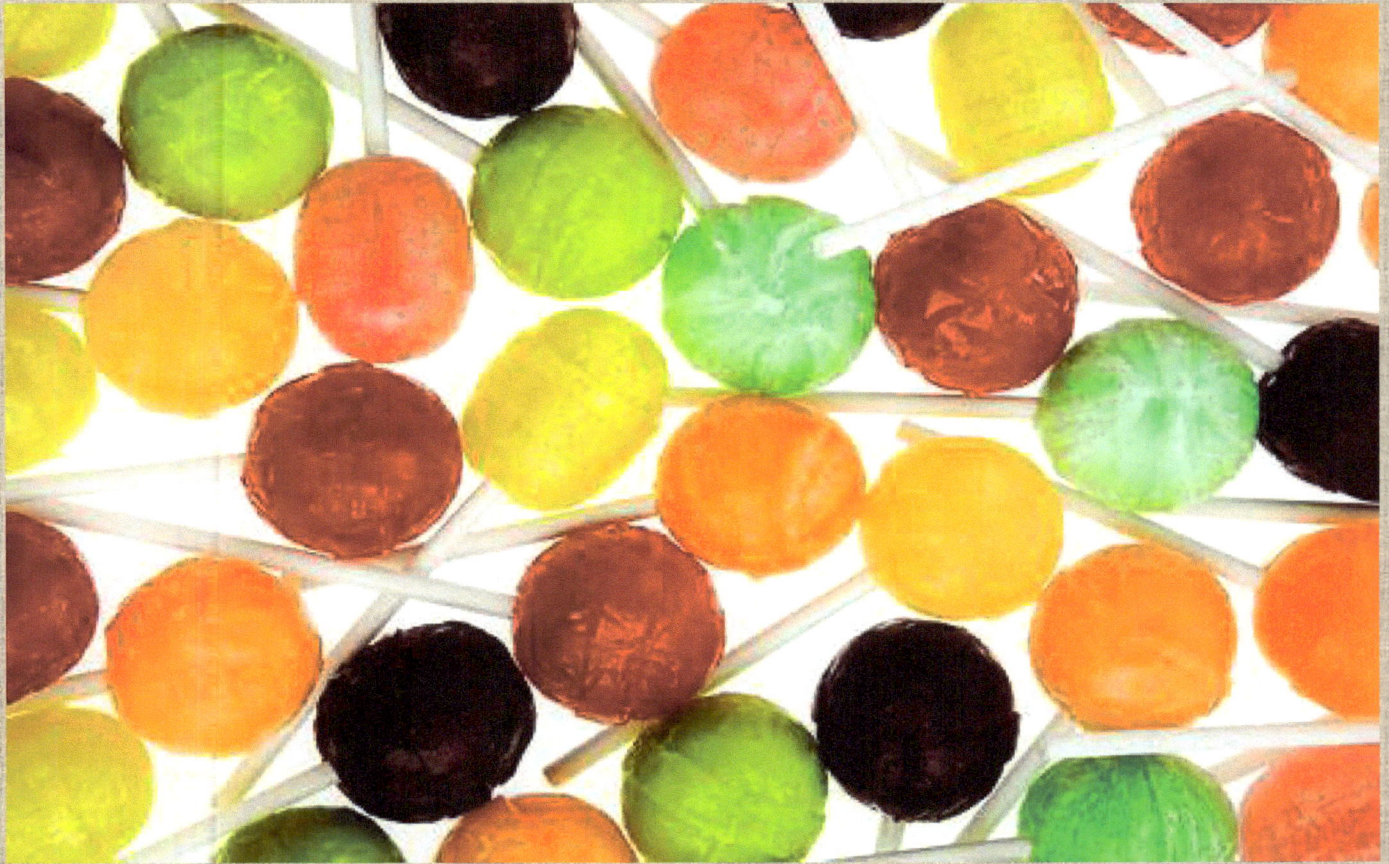

Oranges

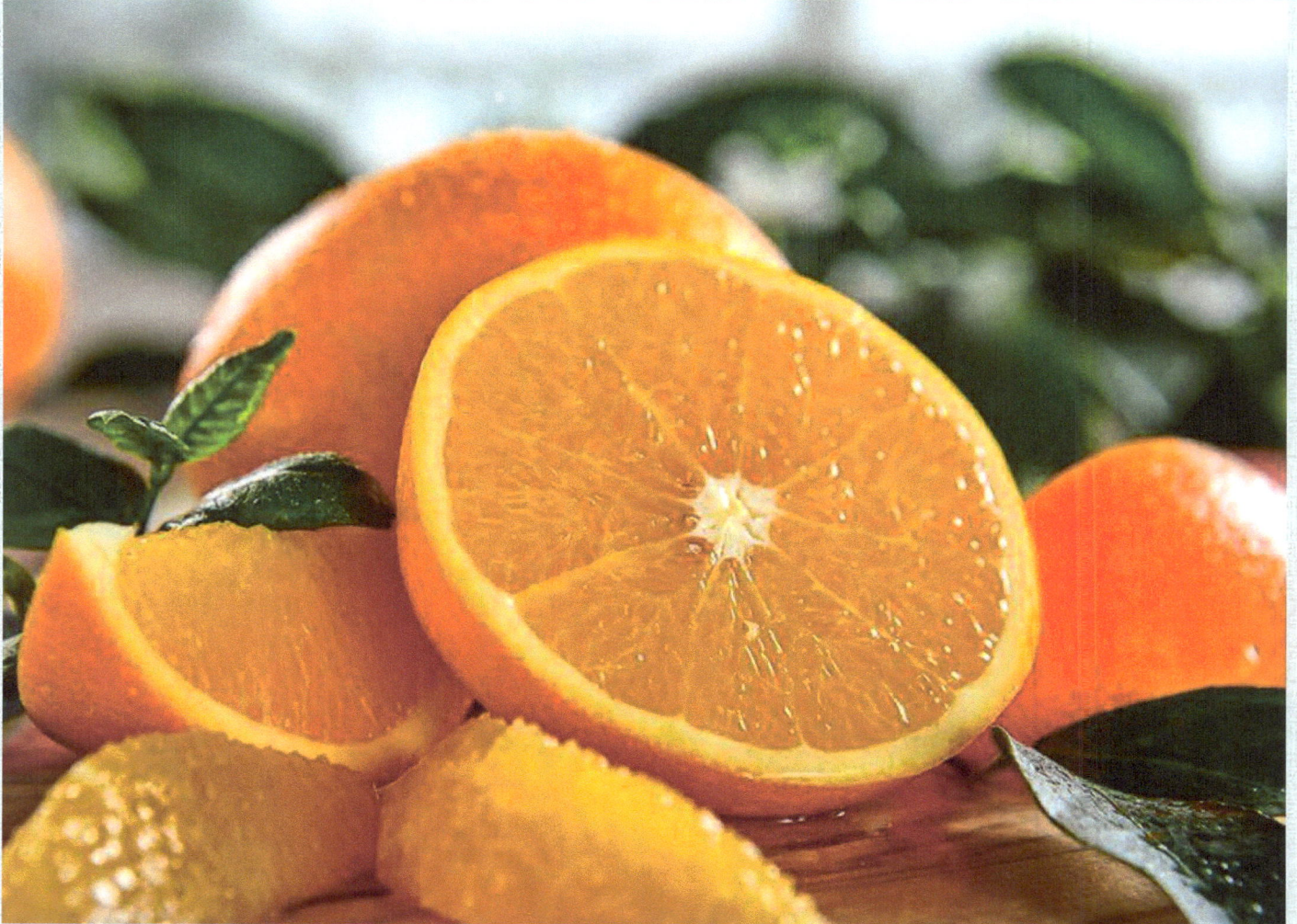

Spinach

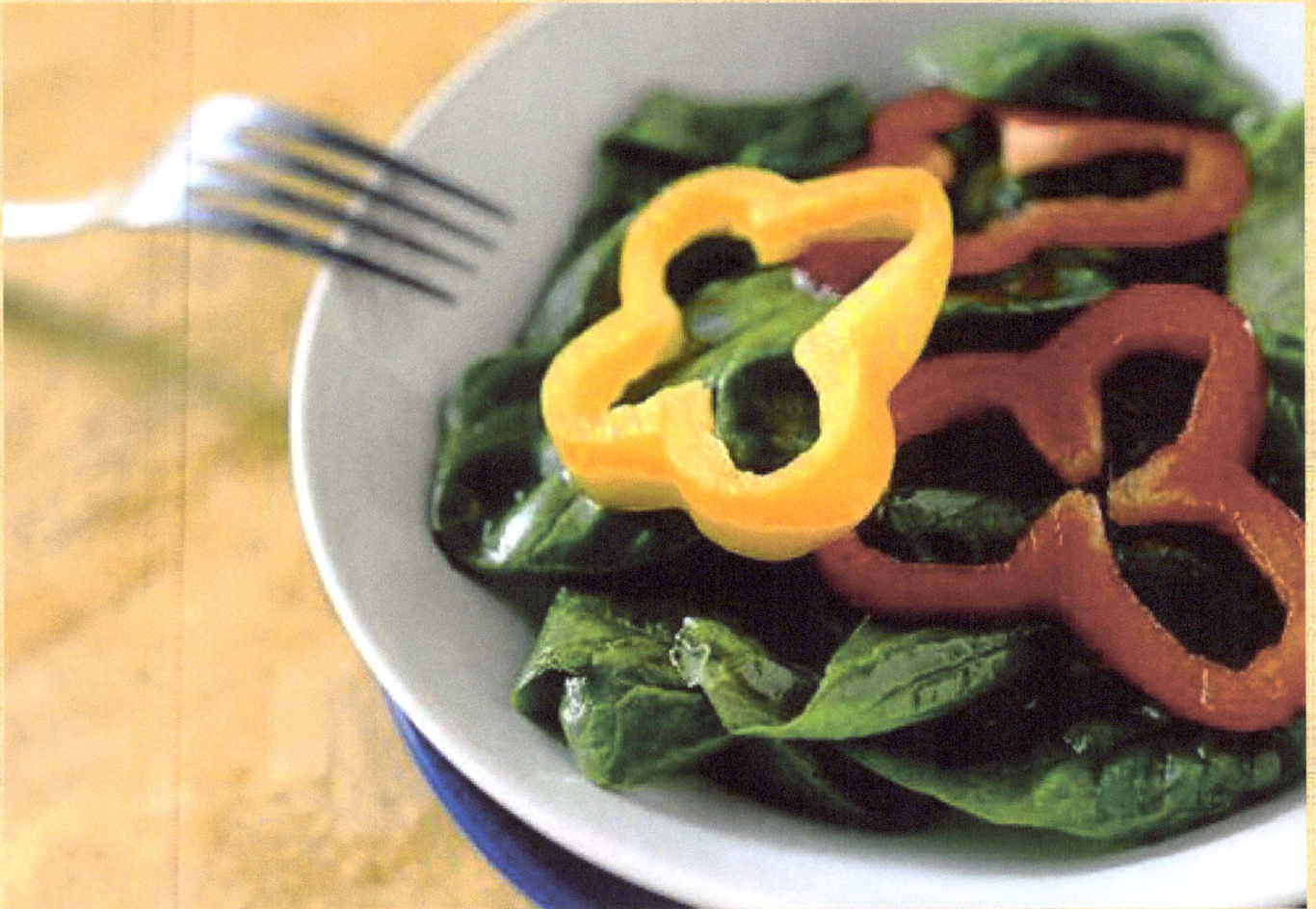

Fatty Fish

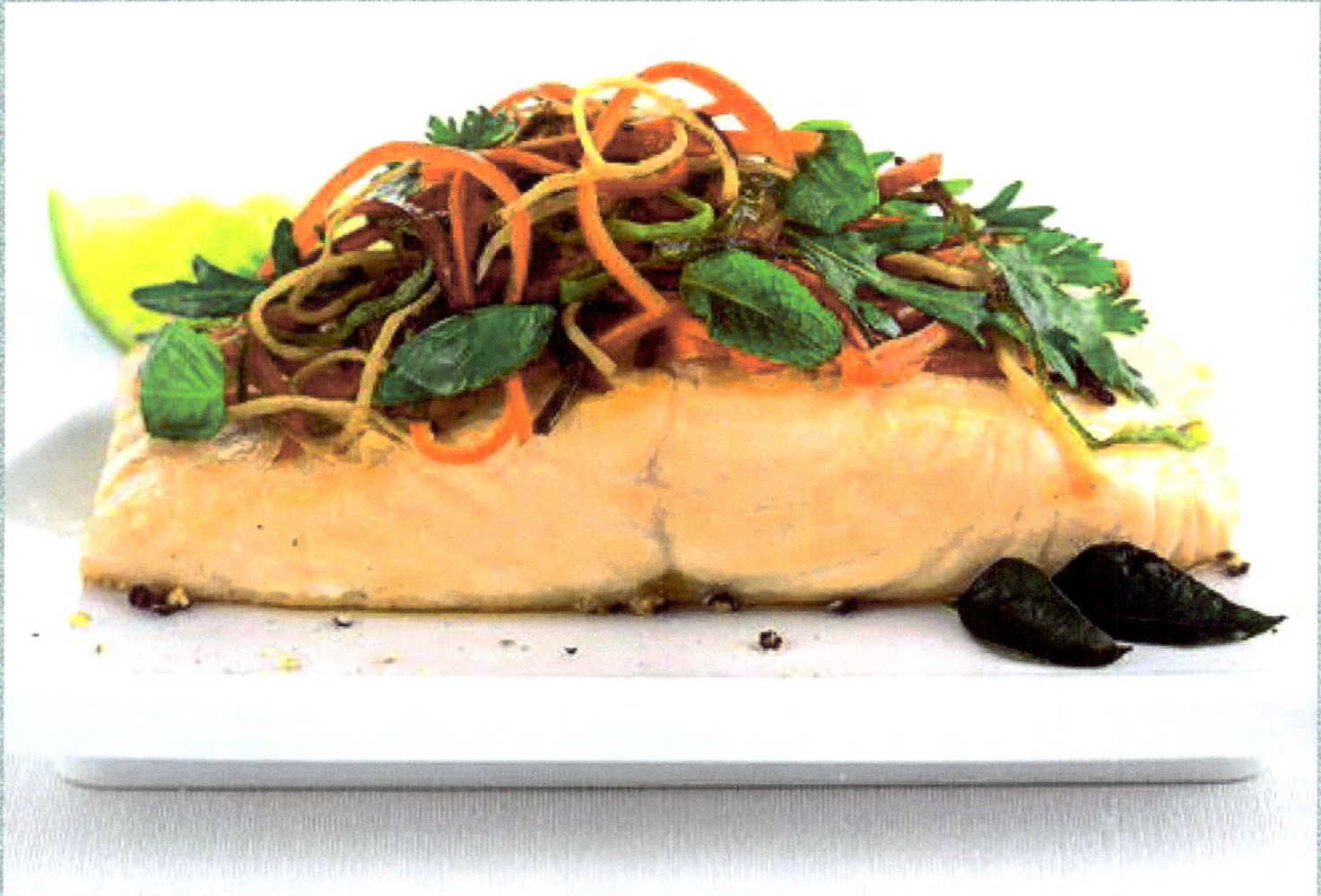

Black Tea

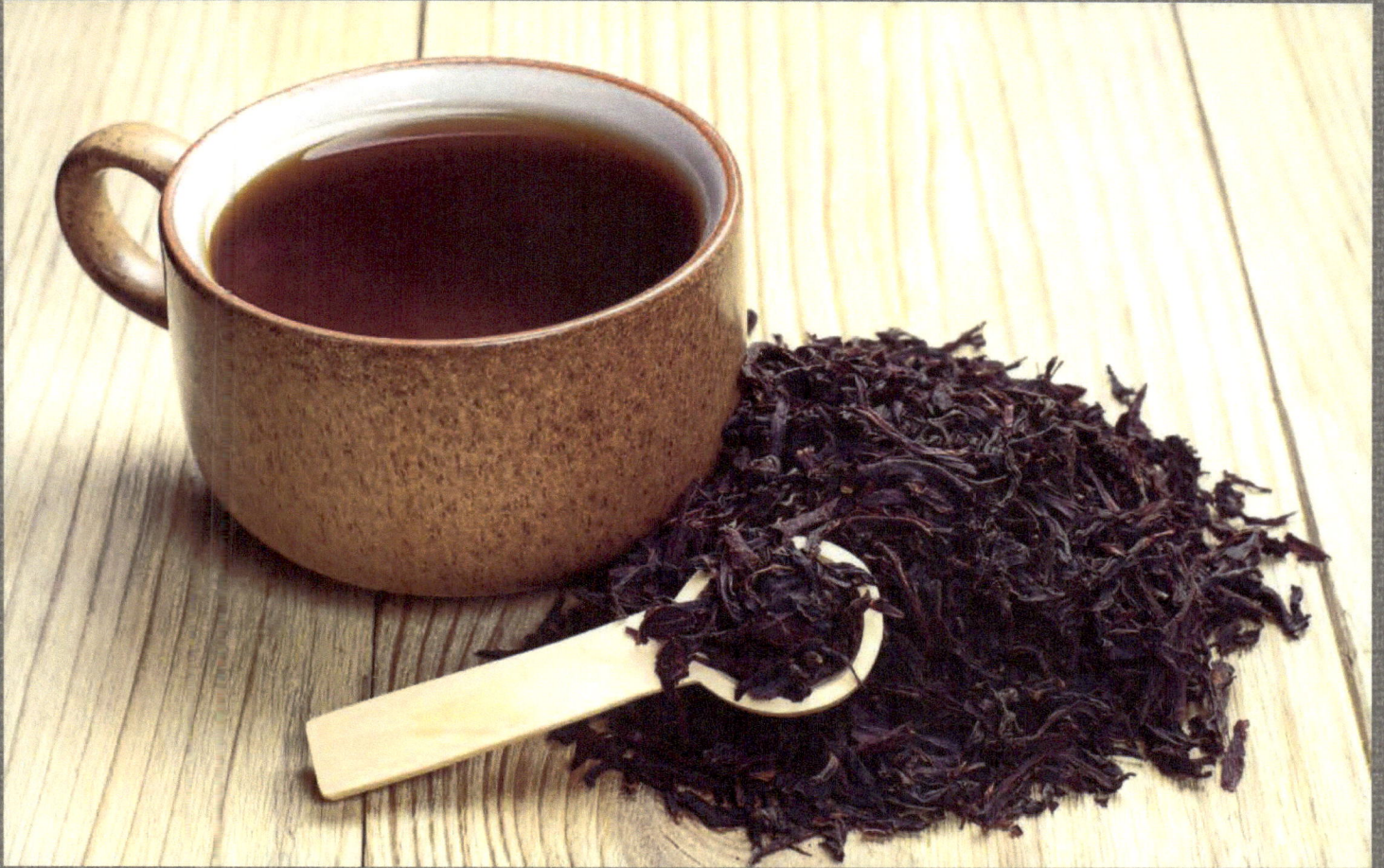

Pistachios

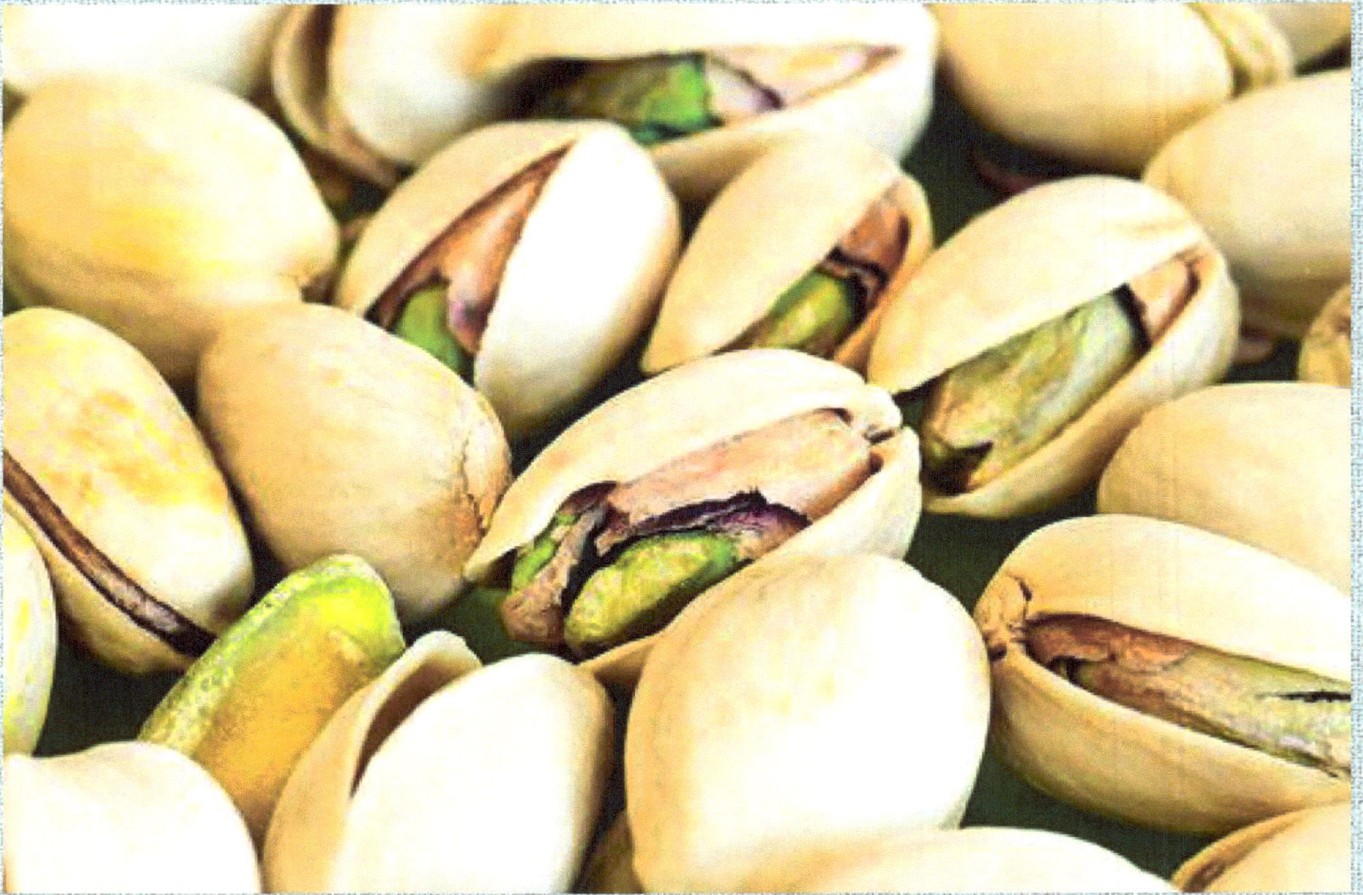

Avocados

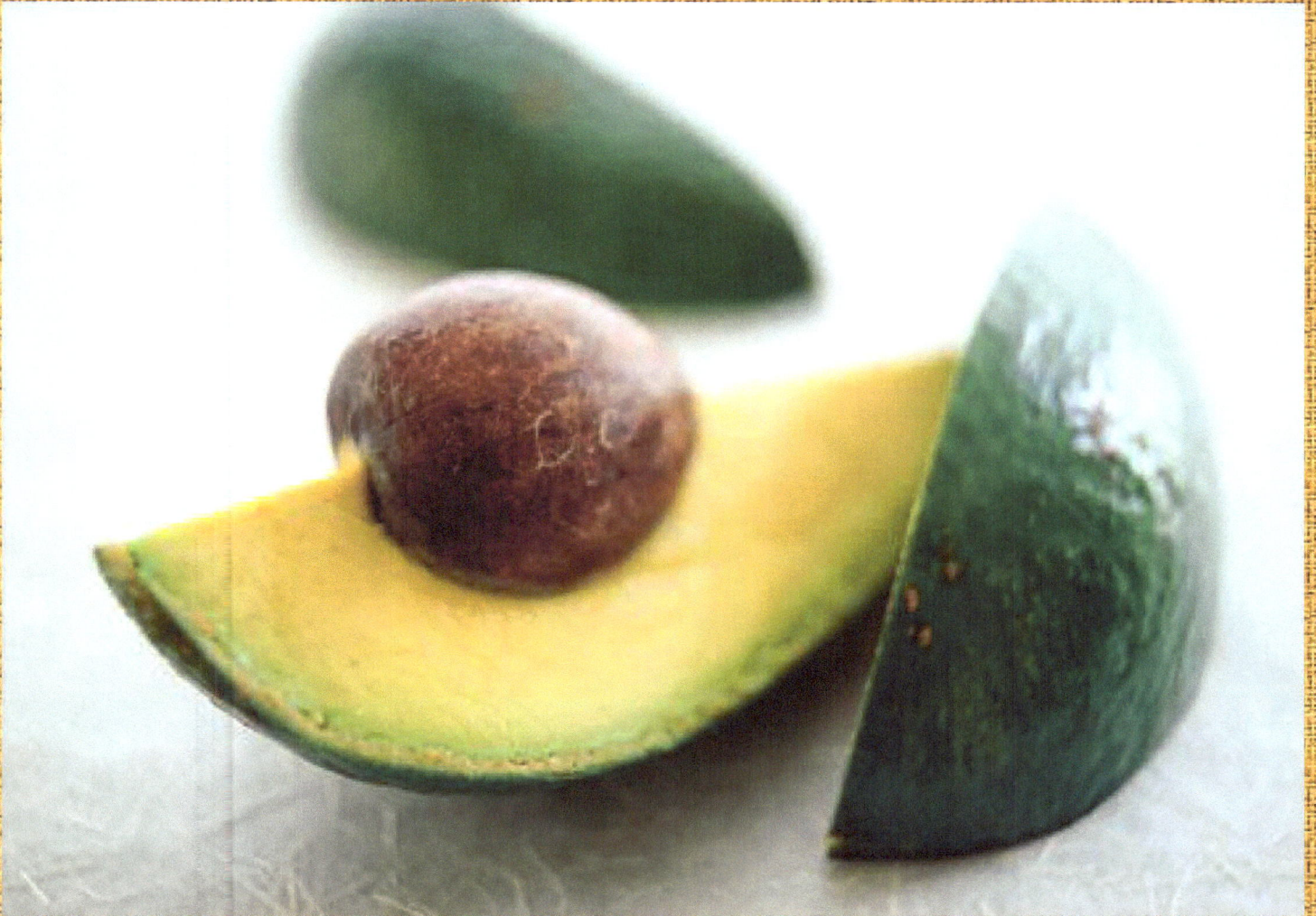

Almonds

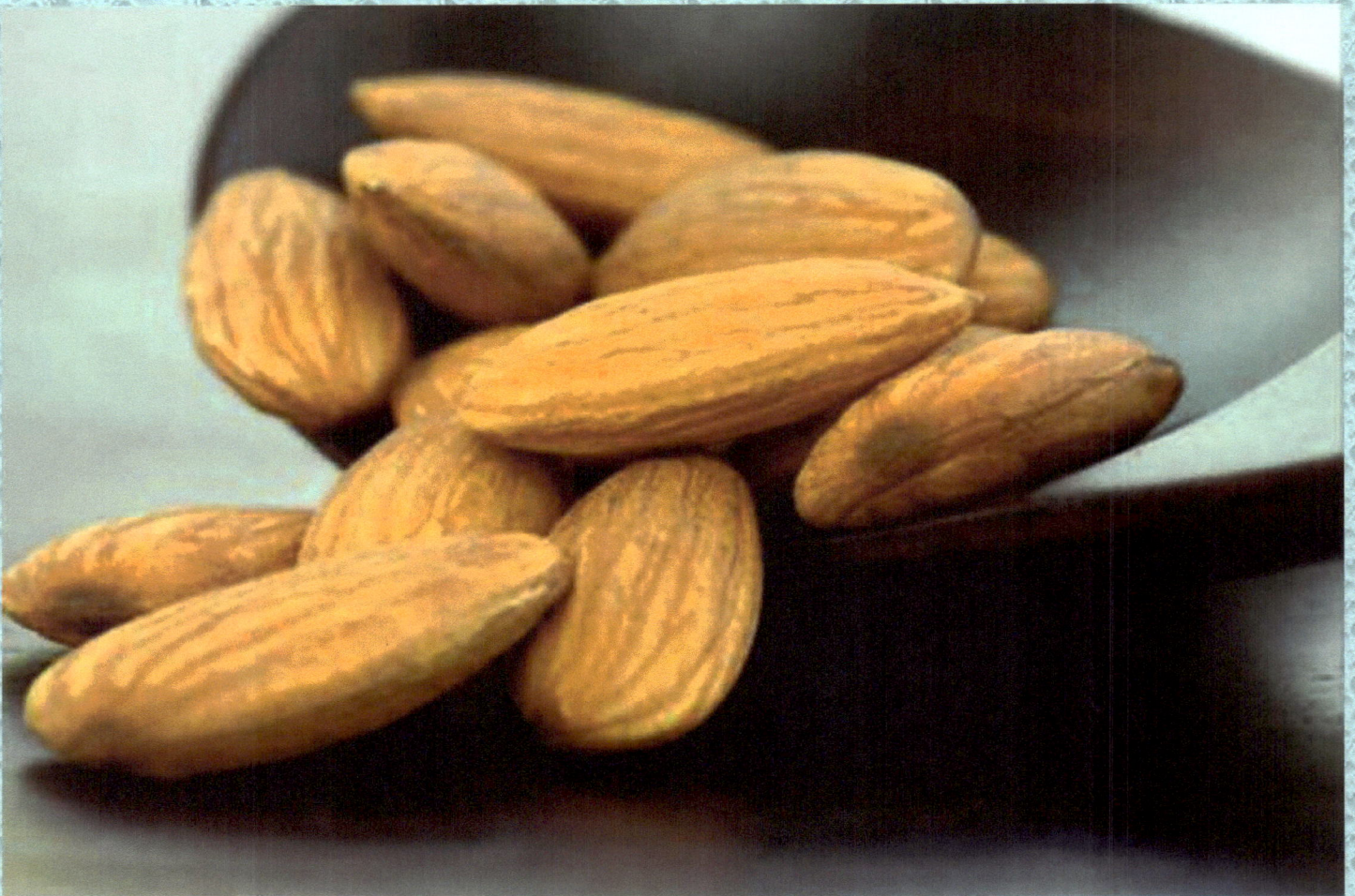

Raw Vegetables

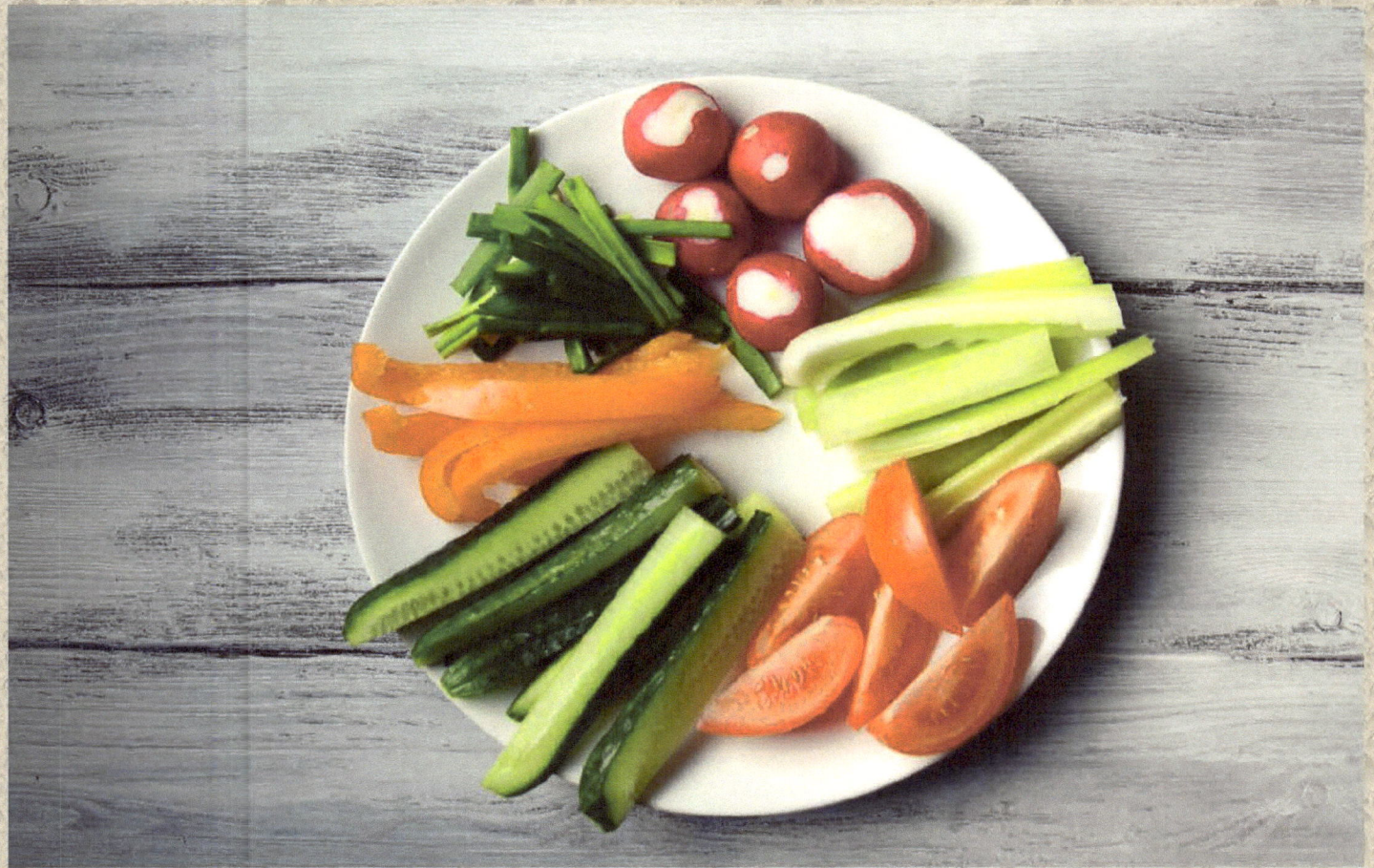

Bedtime Snack

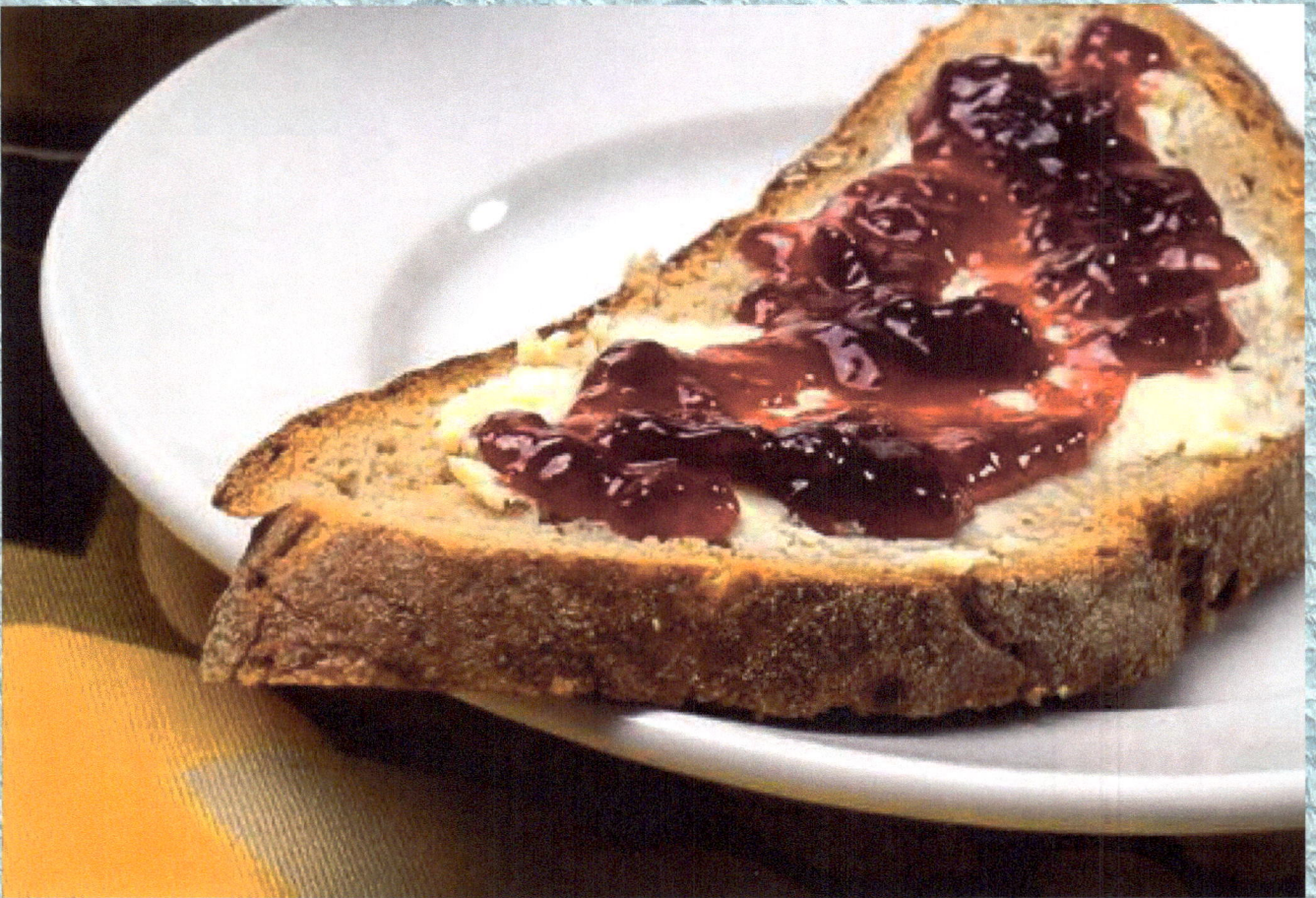

Milk

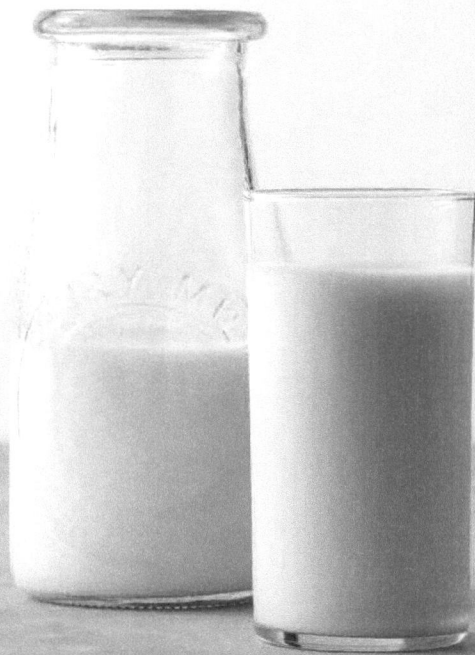

Herbal Supplements

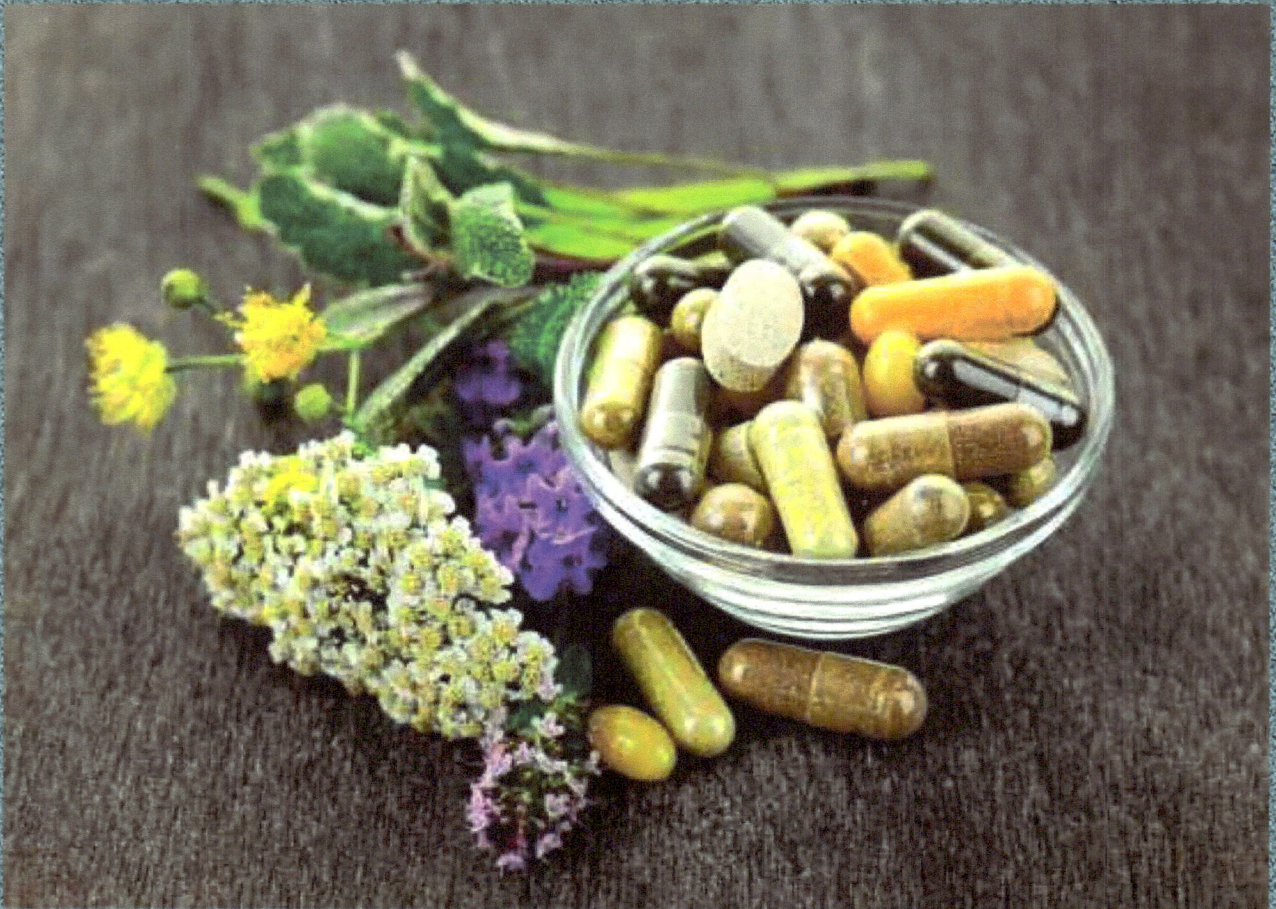

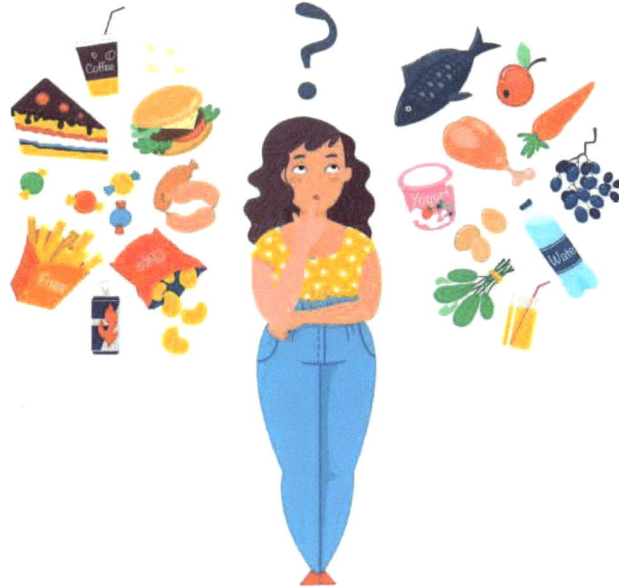

!! MORE ROADBLOCKS TO PROPER
PRENATAL NUTRITION!!

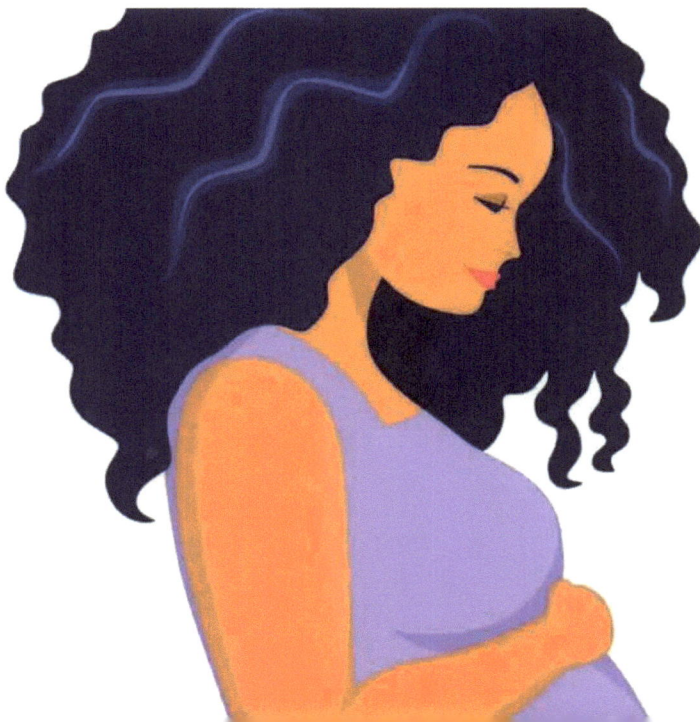

Working

- ❖ Increased Stress

- ❖ Easier to Neglect Nutrition

- ❖ More Fatigue

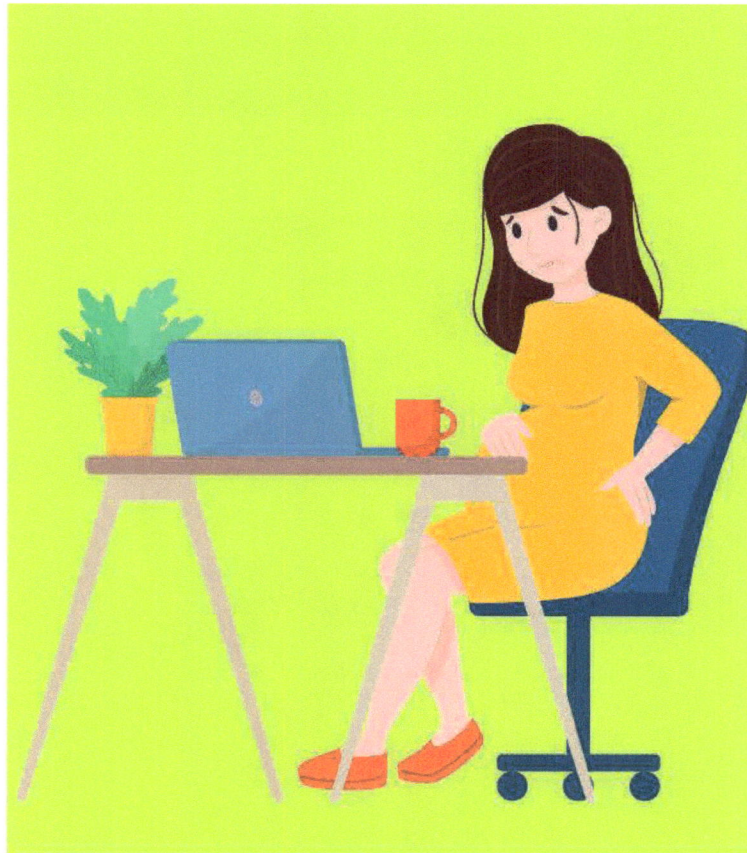

Severe Morning Sickness

- Reduces food consumption

- Loss of Nutrients

- Dehydration Risk

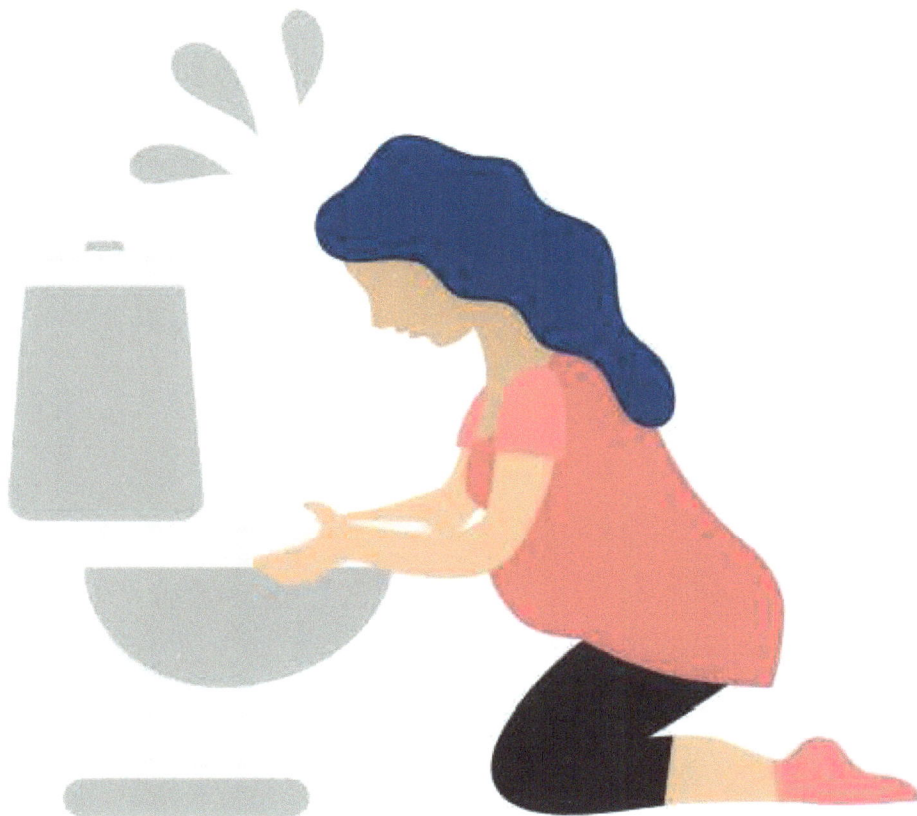

Other Factors:

- **Frequent Eating Out**
  - Can lead to consumption of foods that are not nutrient rich.

- **Very Low Weight Gain During Pregnancy**
  - Could lead to inadequate intake of calories.

- **Very Low or High Pre-Pregnancy Weight**
  - May be a result of poor eating habits.

- **Previous pregnancy**
  - Lowered stores of nutrients in the mother's body.

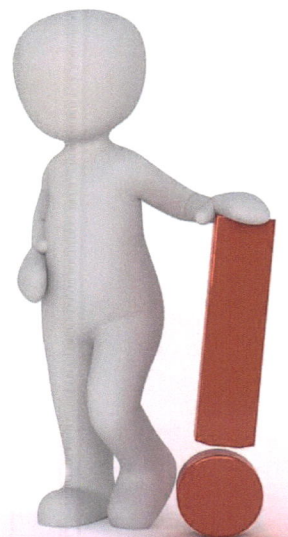

Other Factors (cont):

- **Living Status**
  - Living alone may cause decreased preparation of balanced meals.

- **Frequent Weight Reductionor "Crash Dieting"**
  - May lead to inadequate intake of nutrients.

- **Vegetarian Diet**
  - May lead to inadequate intake of protein and other nutrients.

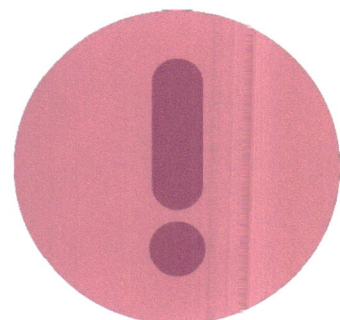

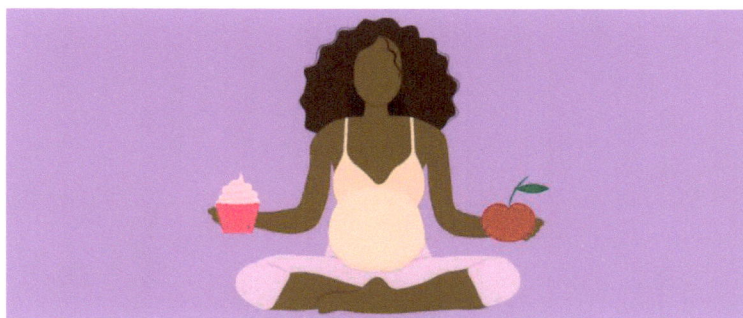

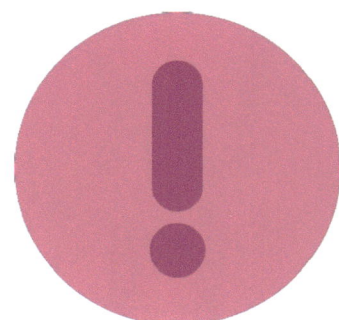

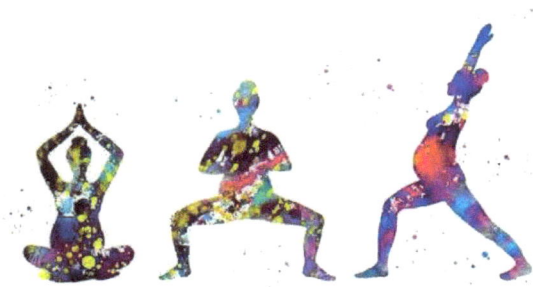

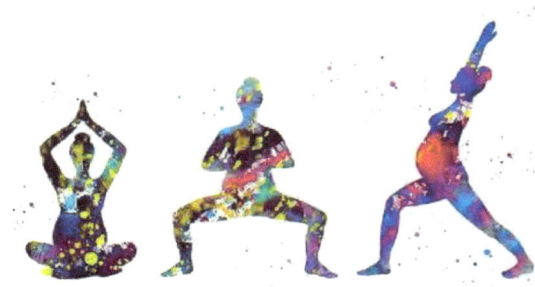

Prenatal Exercise

→ **Regular exercise can be beneficial: Talk to your doctor about your physical activity desires!**

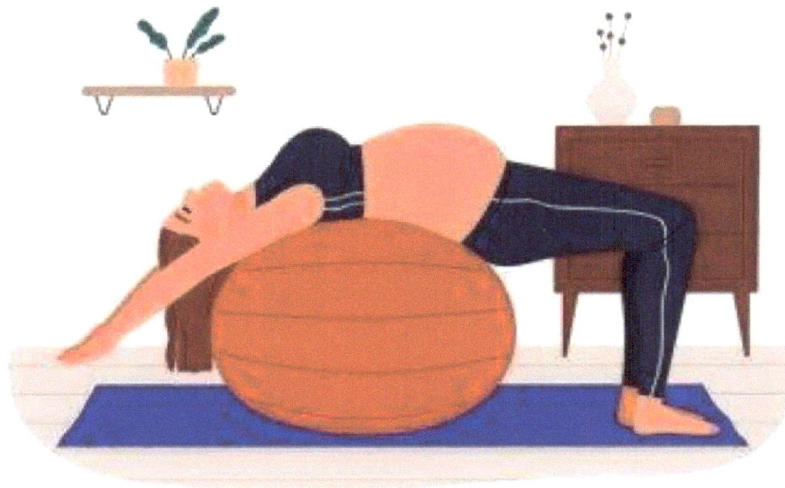

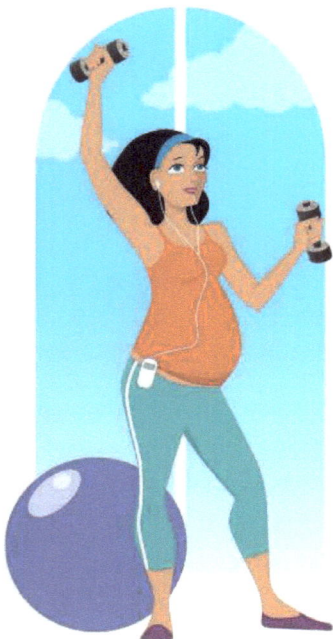

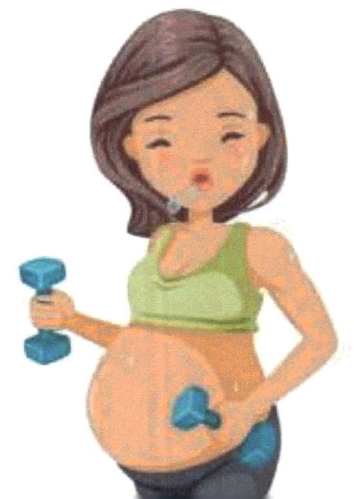

Q & A: Drugs/Alcohol

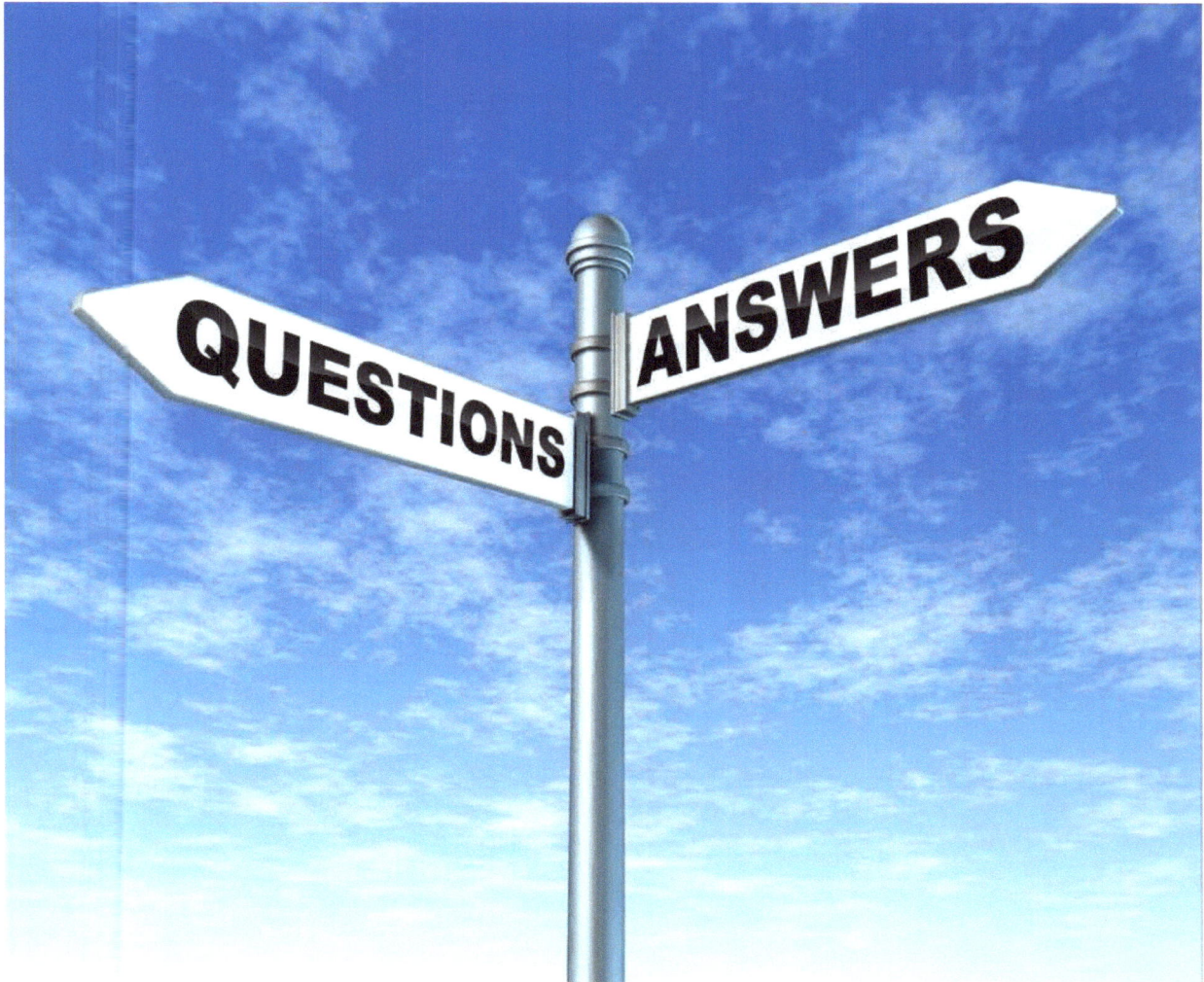

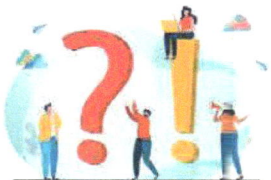

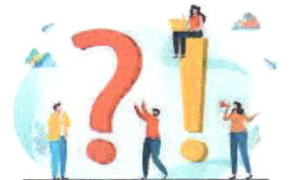

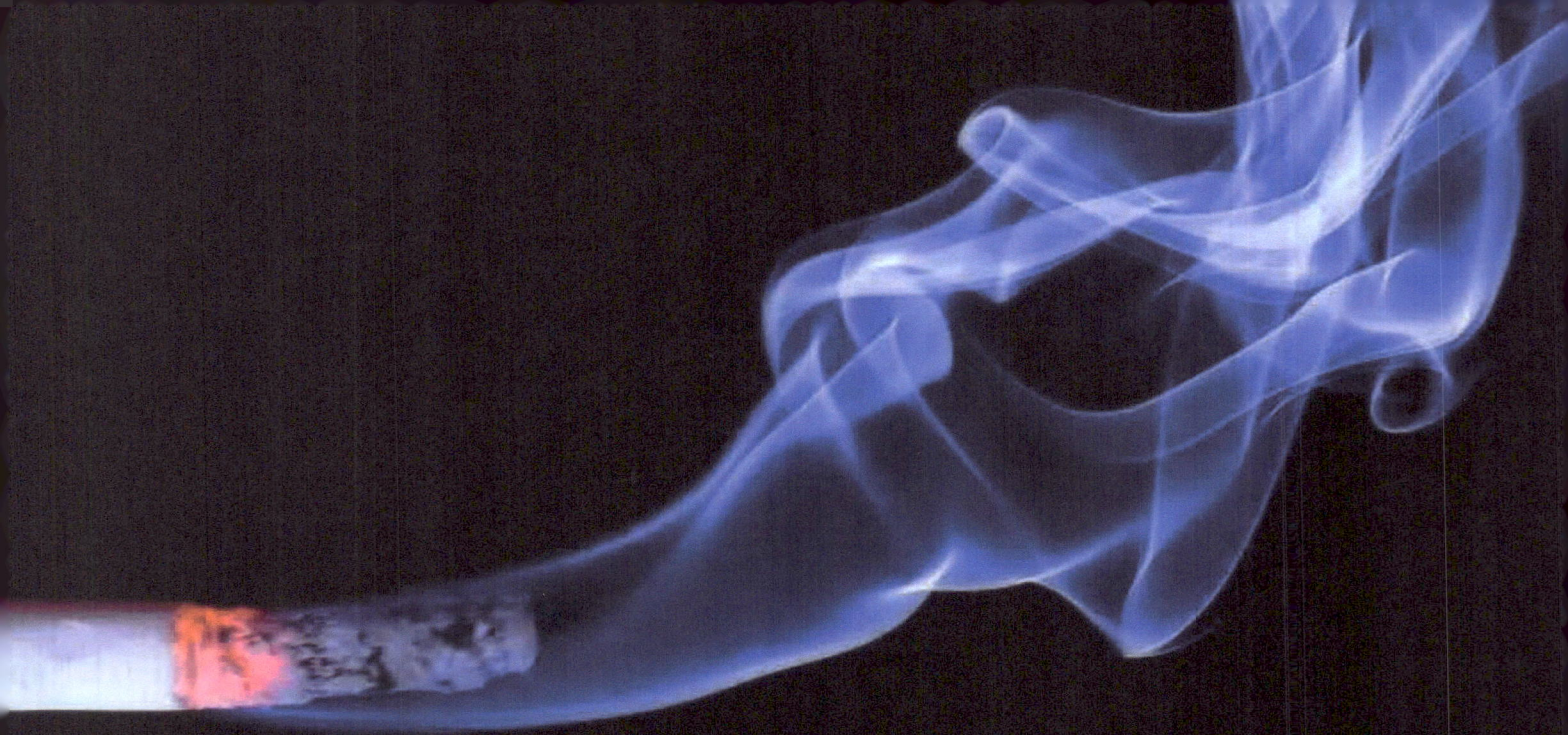

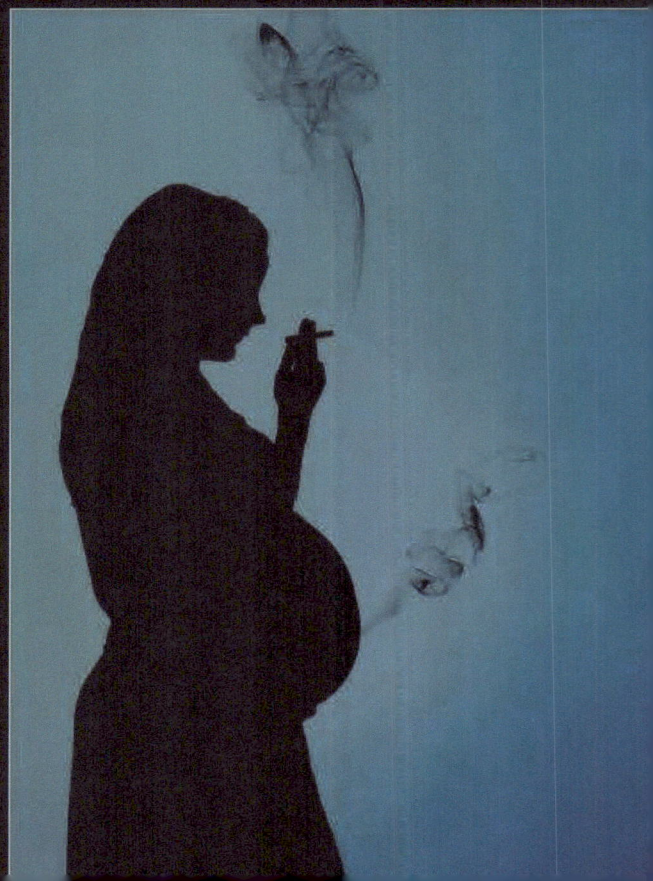

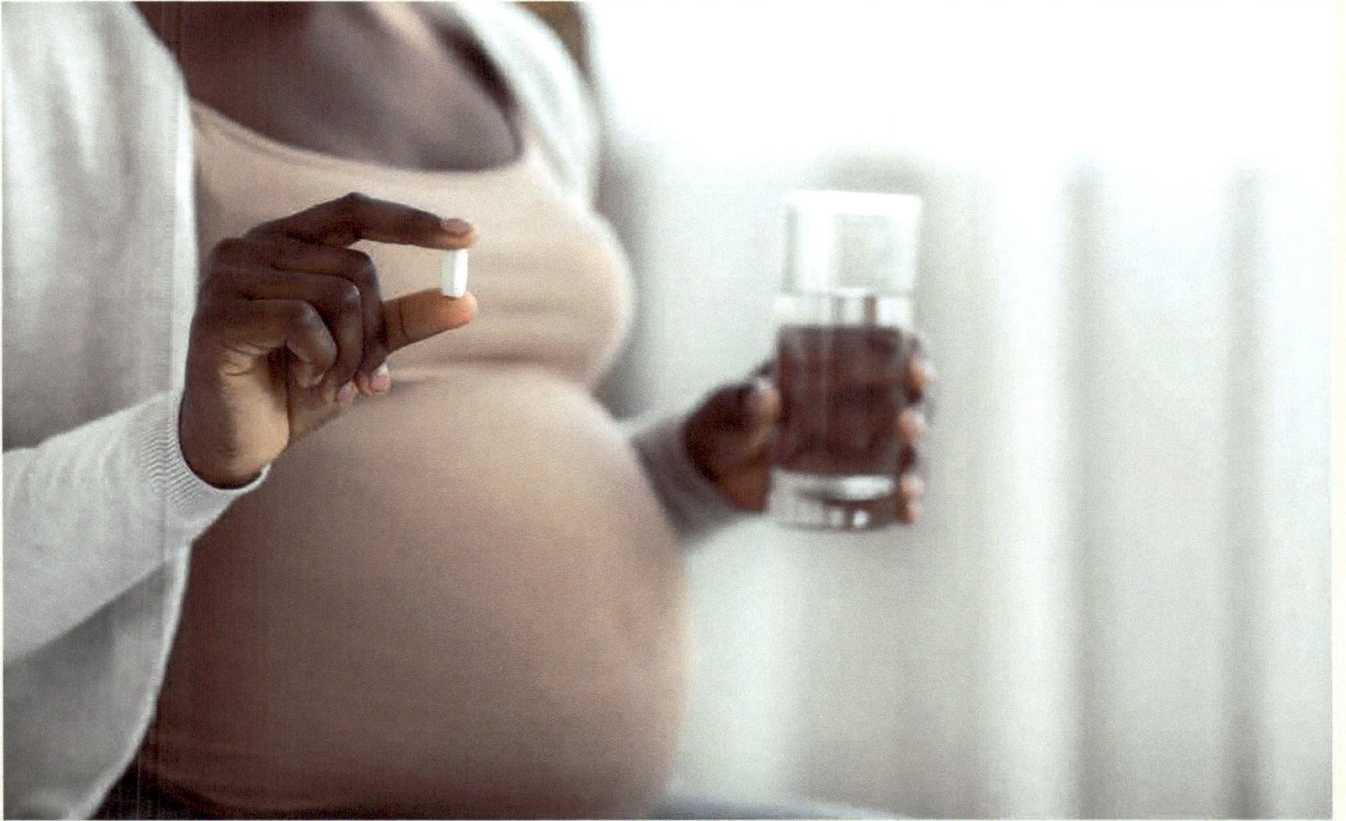

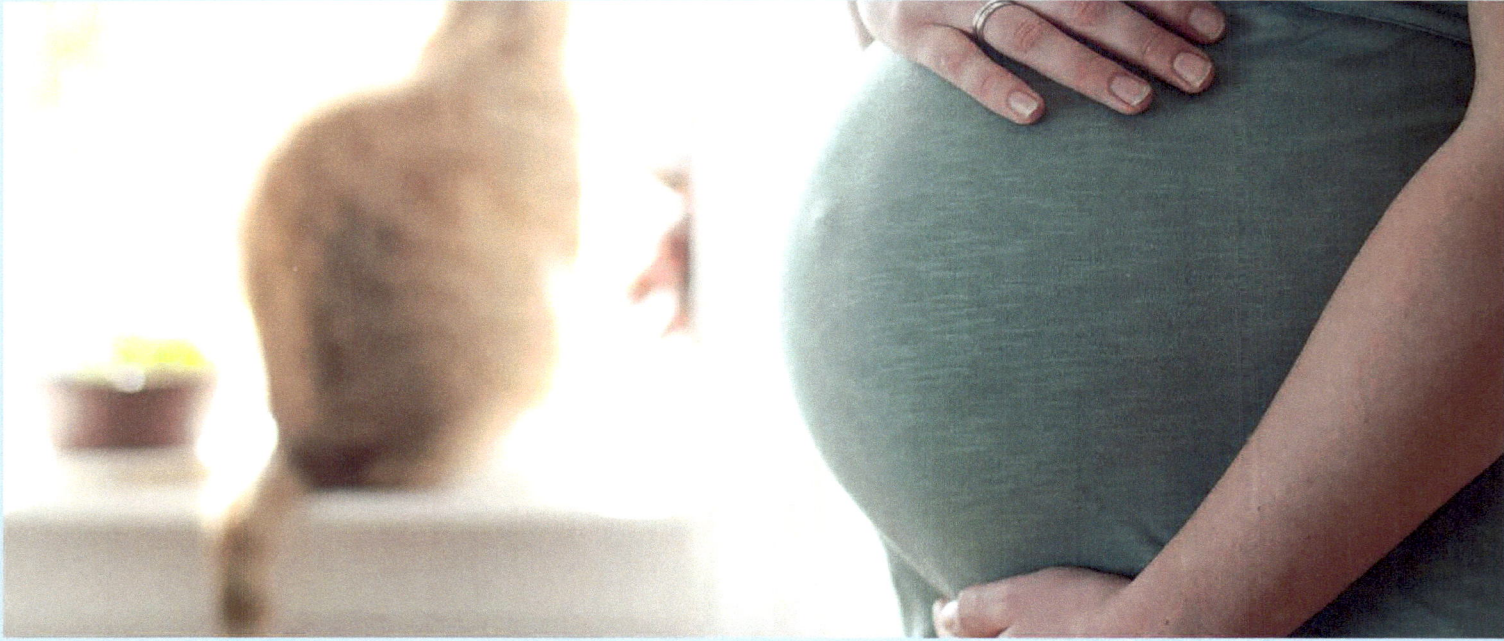
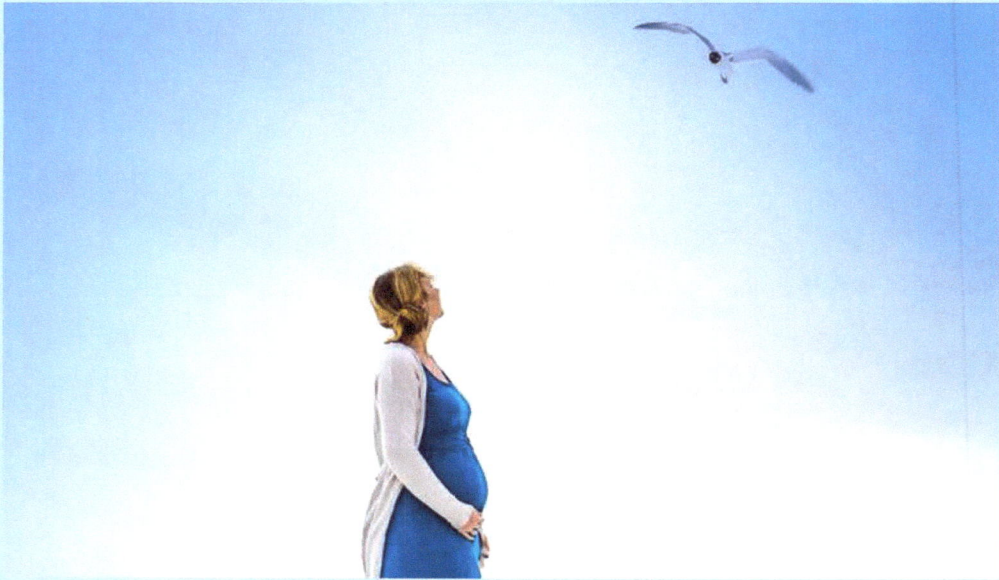

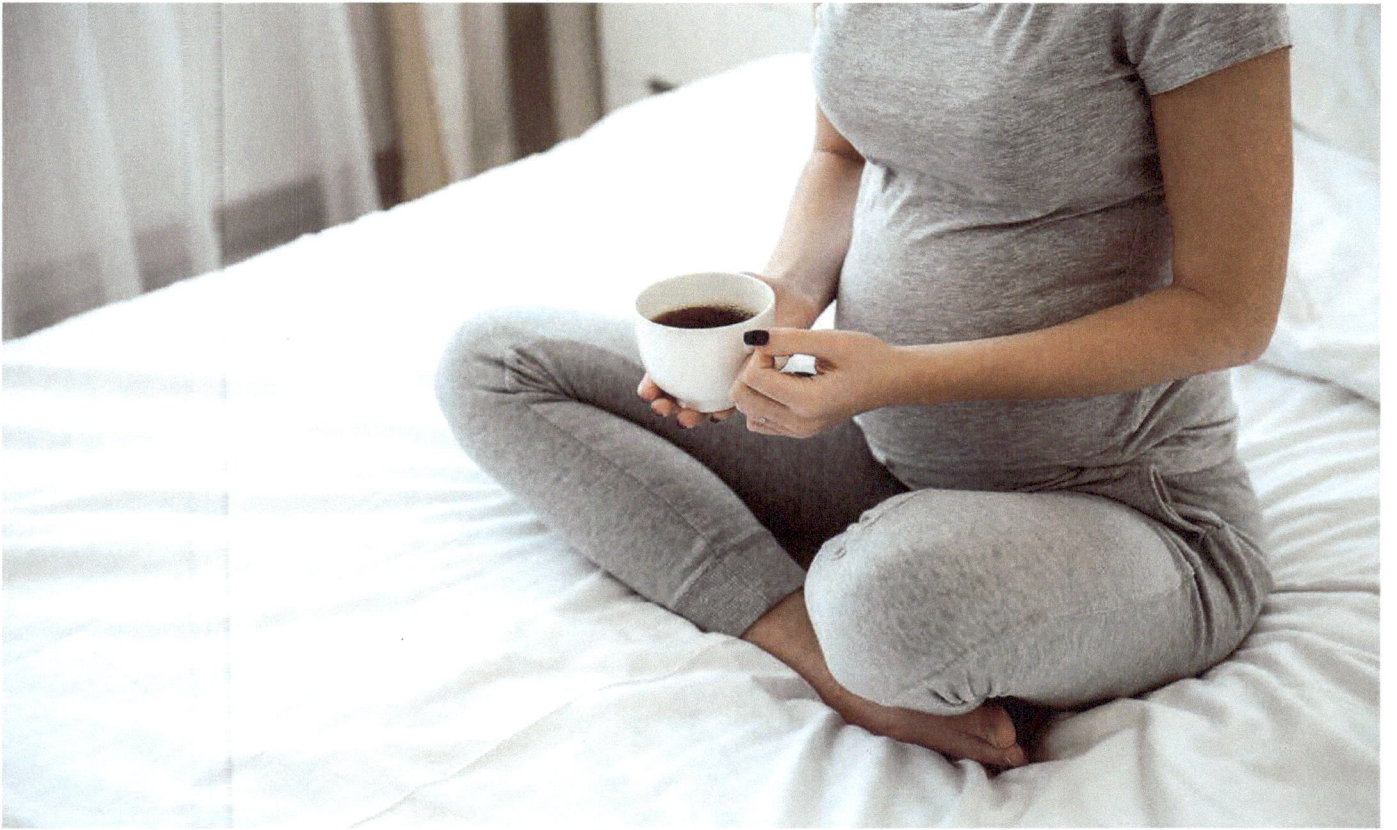

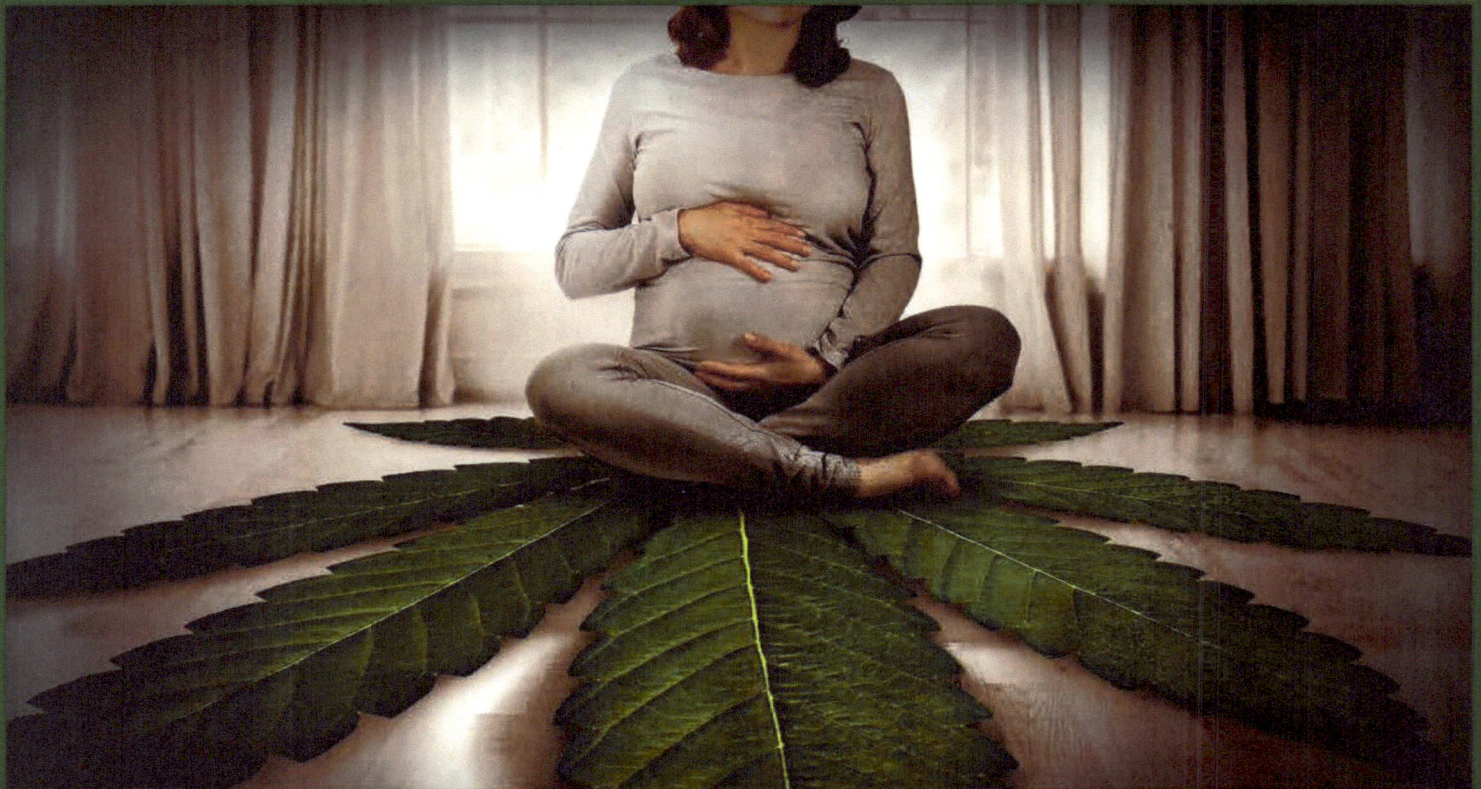

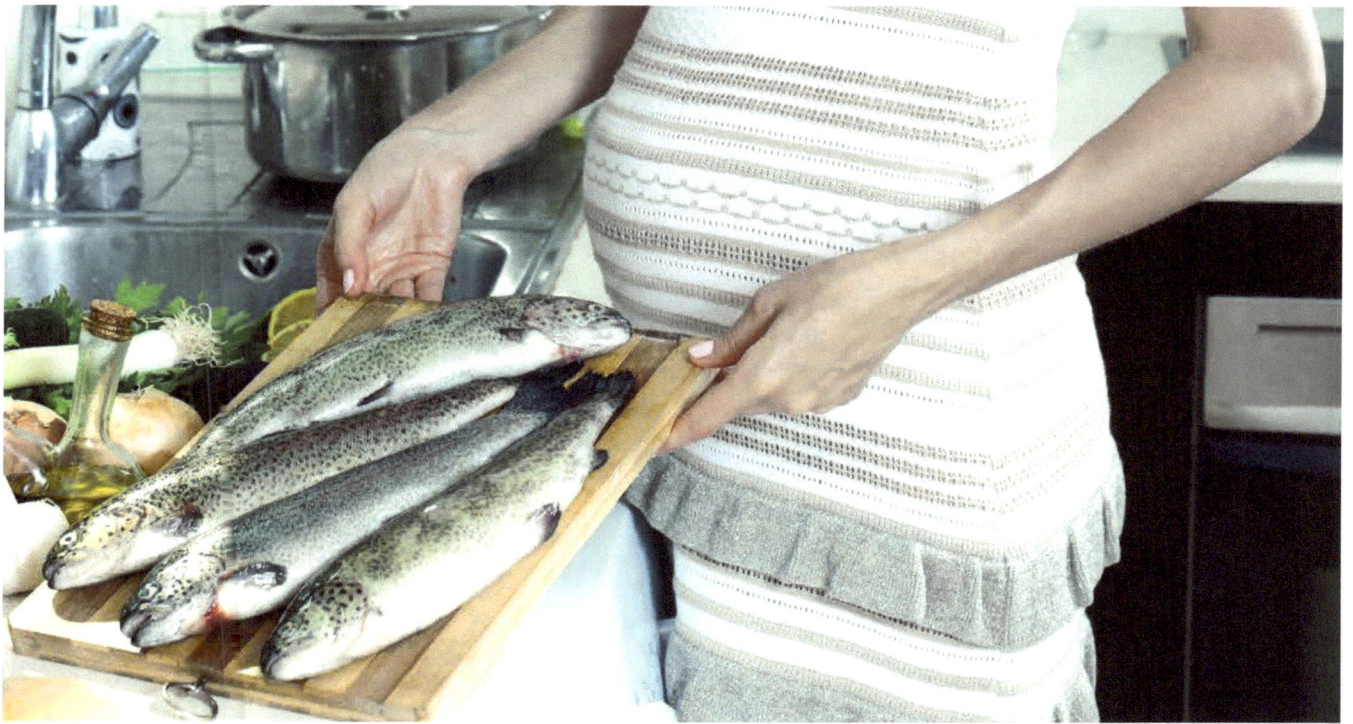

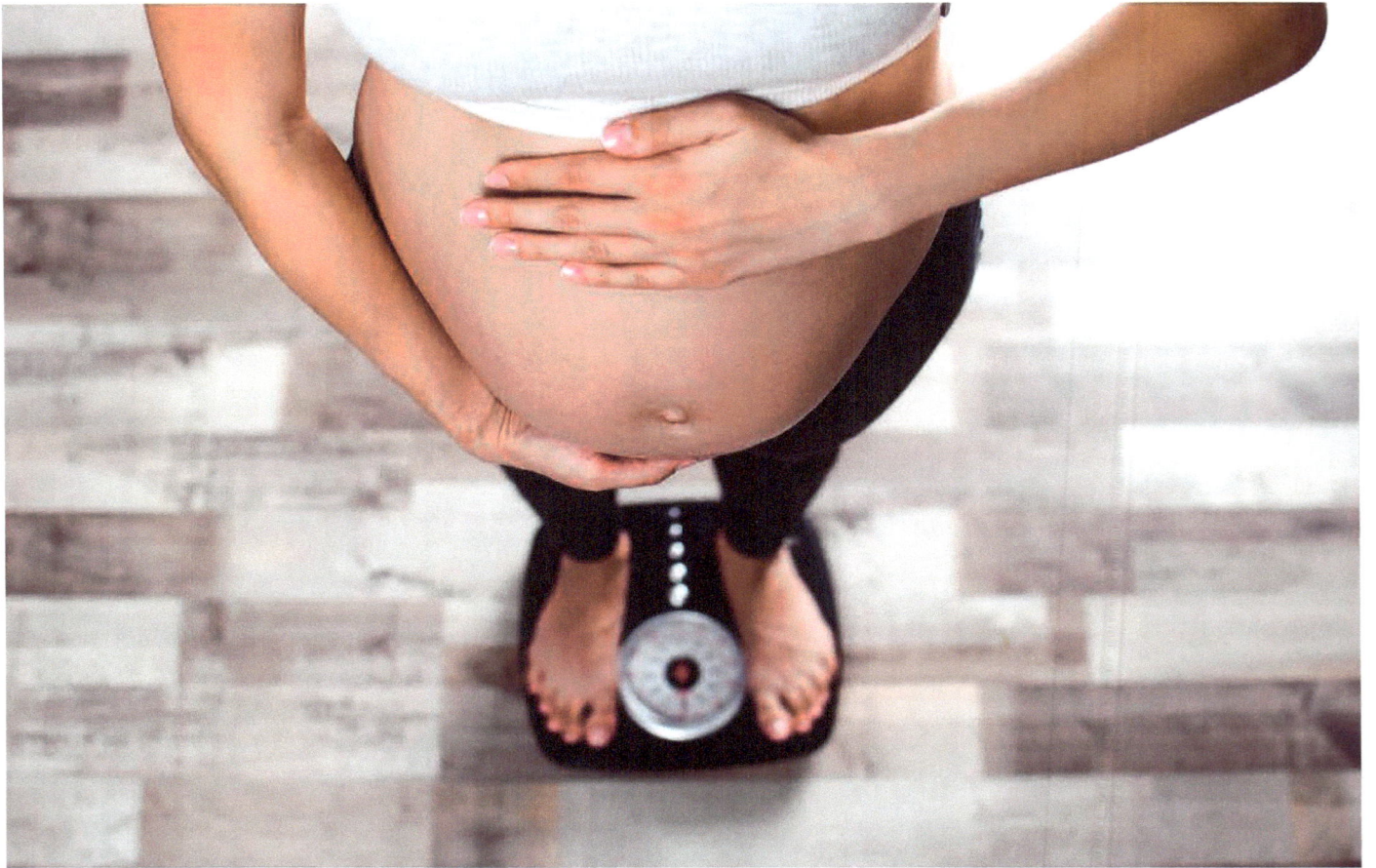

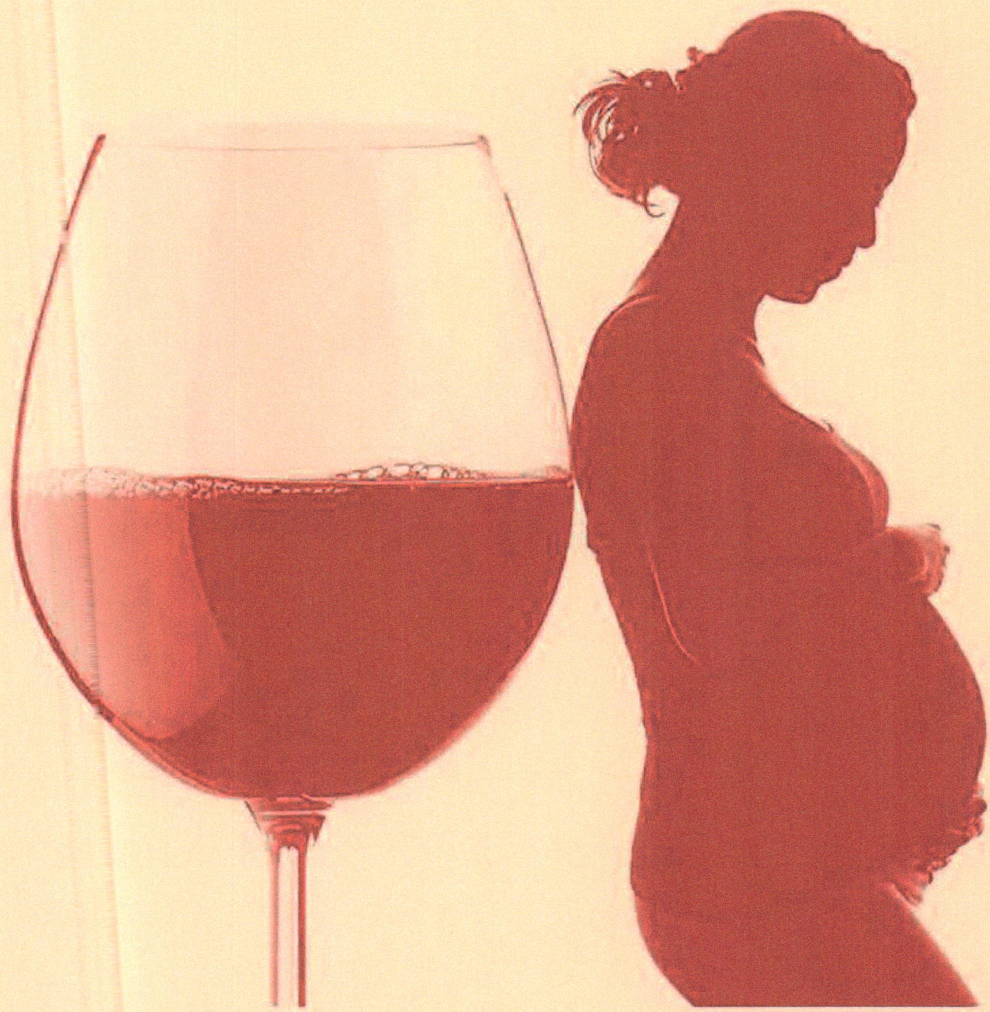

Smoking and Alcohol Use

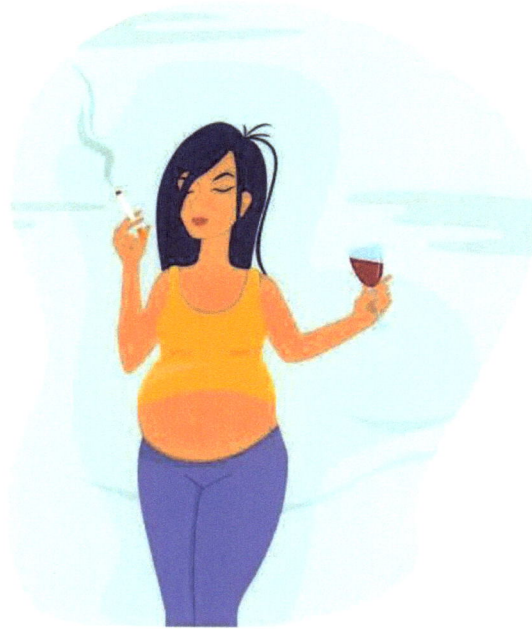

Smoking

➤ Reduces ability to make use of nutrients

➤ Retards taste buds and decreases appetite.

Alcohol Use

➤ Causes inadequate nutrition for mother.

➤ Decreases baby's ability to use nutrients.

How Do I Quit Smoking?

- **Baby and Me Tobacco Free Virtual Program!**
    -Get help to quit tobacco use
    -earn diapers
    -ear wipes
    -earn baby bucks

- **Quit Smoking For Free!**
    www.cdc.gov/tobacco/campaign/tips/quit-smoking/

Smoking during pregnancy can have devastating effects on your baby's development including low birth weight, premature delivery and stillbirth

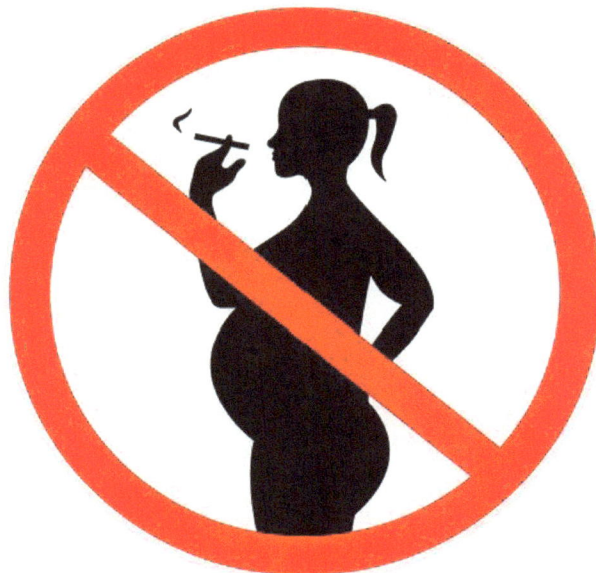

Help for Drug Abuse or Alcoholism

- **How can you get help to quit using street drugs and alcohol?**

- Talk to your health care provider. They can help you get treatment to quit.

- Or contact:
- National Council on Alcoholism and Drug Dependence (800) 622-2255

- Substance Abuse Treatment Facility Locator (800) 662-4357

- Contact the Women's Recovery Center in Xenia, OH (937) 562-2400

*Drinking Alcohol During Pregnancy is
the leading cause of preventable mental retardation*

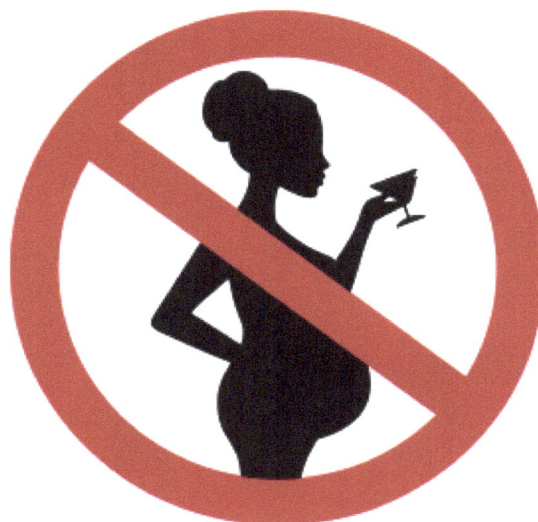

Key Takeaways:

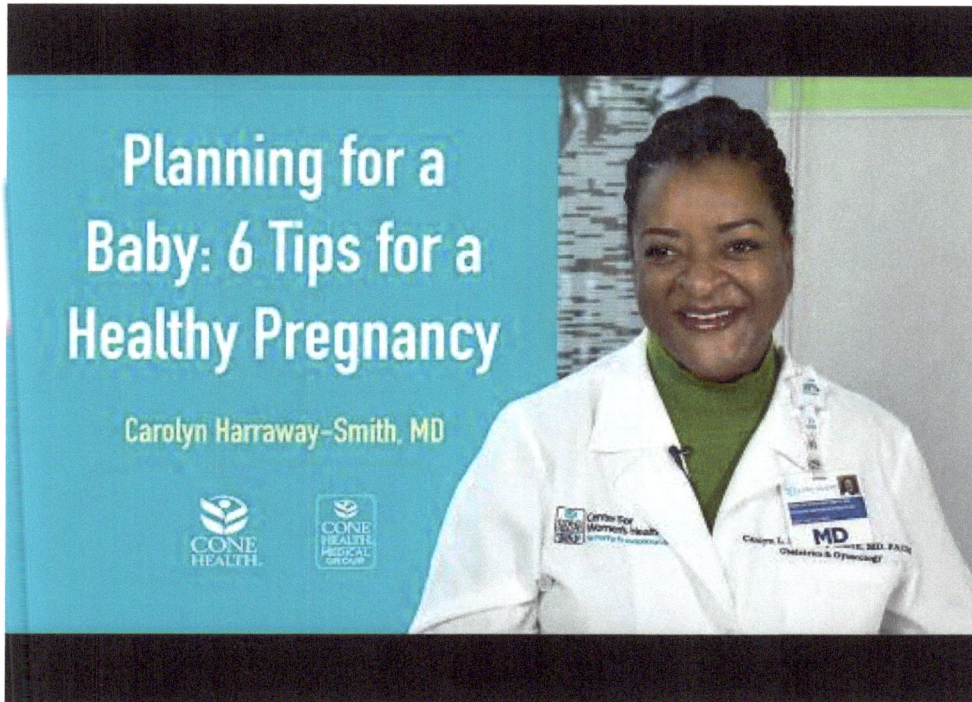

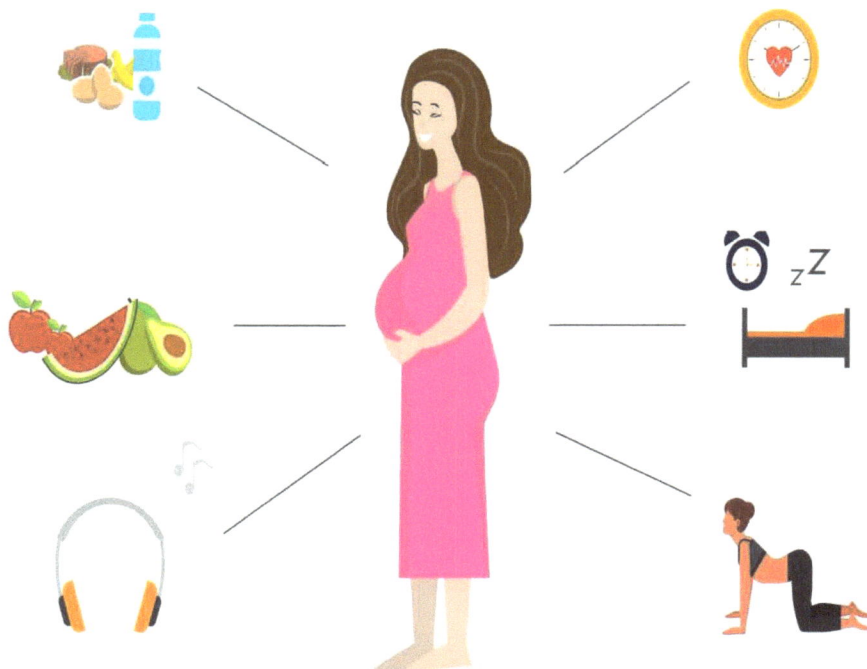

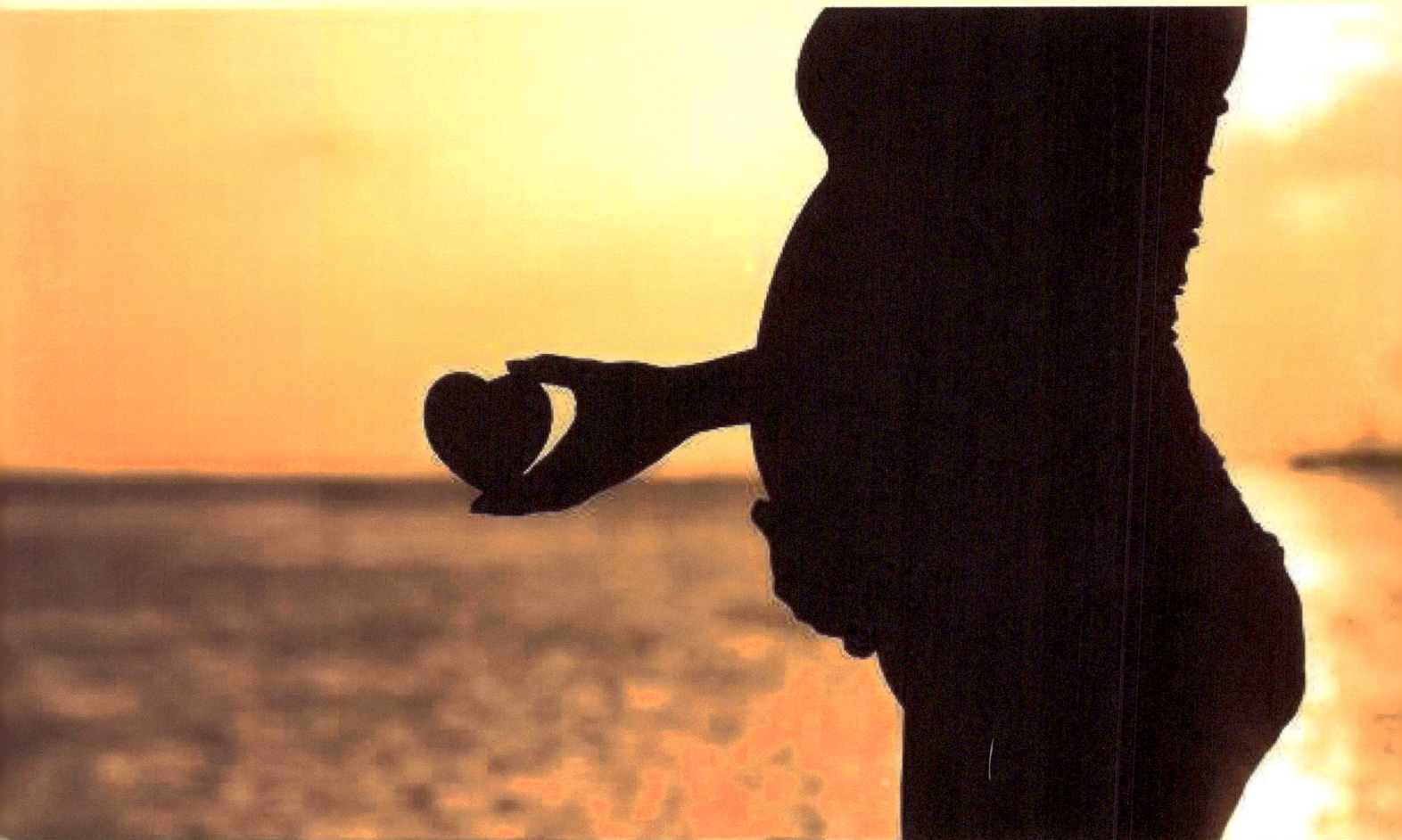

Embrace the Journey!